Managing Change in
Healthcare
Using Action Research

Paul Parkin

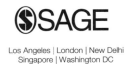

Los Angeles | London | New Delhi
Singapore | Washington DC

First published 2009

Reprinted 2010

SAGE Publications Ltd
1 Oliver's Yard
55 City Road
London EC1Y 1SP

SAGE Publications Inc.
2455 Teller Road
Thousand Oaks, California 91320

SAGE Publications India Pvt Ltd
B 1/I 1 Mohan Cooperative Industrial Area
Mathura Road
New Delhi 110 044

SAGE Publications Asia-Pacific Pte Ltd
33 Pekin Street #02-01
Far East Square
Singapore 048763

Library of Congress Control Number: 2008929611

British Library Cataloguing in Publication data

A catalogue record for this book is available from the British Library

ISBN 978-1-4129-2258-6
ISBN 978-1-4129-2259-3 (pbk)

Typeset by C&M Digitals Pvt Ltd, Chennai, India
Printed and bound in Great Britain by CPI Antony Rowe, Chippenham, Wiltshire
Printed on paper from sustainable resources

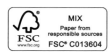

Managing Change in
Healthcare
Using Action Research

For my parents, Dynely and Bobby Parkin

Contents

Acknowledgements

I wish to express my appreciation to those who have patiently supported me in this venture:

From SAGE: Alison Poyner for starting the process, Anna Luker, and especially Zoë Elliott-Fawcett for her continuous advice and encouragement.

To the anonymous reviewers who have endured my attempts at refinement: resolute writers can be changed by their suggestions.

To work colleagues at Brunel University who covered my absences.

To Brunel students attending 'Managing Contemporary Practice' and 'Managing People at Work' courses for their contributions and encouragement.

Lastly, to my wife Jenny Parkin, who has diligently and uncomplainingly proof-read every word and cross-checked every reference.

Any remaining errors are my responsibility entirely.

List of Abbreviations

BMA	British Medical Association
CD	Community Development
CPD	Continuous Professional Development
CPF	Clinical Practice Facilitator
CS	Clinical Supervision
DCA	Department of Constitutional Affairs
DH	Department of Health
DHSS	Department of Health and Social Security
DLP	Daily Living Plan
GP	General Practitioner
HODU	Haematology-Oncology Day Unit
NHS	National Health Service
NICE	National Institute of Clinical Excellence
PAR	Participatory Action Research
PCO	Primary Care Organization
P-CGP	Patient-Centred Goal Planning
PCS	Primary Care Services
PEST	Political, Economic, Social, Technical
RCT	Randomized Clinical Trial
SWOT	Strengths, Weaknesses, Opportunities, Threats

It is possible to change the world, but impossible without the
mobilization of the dominated

Paulo Freire
(*Letters to Cristina: Reflections on my Life and Work*,
New York: Routledge. 1996: 183)

1

Introduction: Setting the Scene

Healthcare: a changing environment

Healthcare provision in Britain is dominated by the National Health Service (NHS). Its size, the scope and extent of its services, the range, levels and diverse skills of its workforce and its unique position in the political system, makes it unlike any other organization in the United Kingdom. It is reported to be the 5th largest organization in the world (Carvel, 2005) employing over 1.3 million staff (Winterton, 2004). Many parts of the service, such as local hospitals, specialist services, staff groups, and General Practice (GP) surgeries are known to have a unique and special place in the hearts and minds of the public (Klein, 1999; Smith, 2002). Hjul (2006) argues that GPs, as the public face of healthcare, are more likely to be known by people, who refer to them as 'their' doctor, than any other public servant.

The NHS was created by a Labour administration in the post-war policy drive of 'nationalization' where the state extended its powers of control to major infrastructure industries and has been considered a cornerstone of the British welfare state since its inception in 1948 (Salauroo and Burnes, 1998). The road and rail services were nationalized in the same year the NHS was created; electricity in 1946; coal in 1947; iron, steel and gas in 1949. All these services have, often in the name of efficiency, now been privatized, broken up or given quasi-independency. Except, that is, the NHS, leading a *Sunday Times* editorial to claim that it has:

> trundled along as an inefficient, centrally run command and control model that would be more at home in North Korea than a supposedly modern western economy. (*Sunday Times*, 2003: 18)

During its lifetime its principles have endured, however, the guiding policies, organization and delivery of health services have been subjected to continual reforms. The focus of changes in the NHS depend on the orientations and philosophies of its political masters and involve everything from the macro level of funding, service planning and delivery to the micro level of personal care and ward cleanliness.

For all organizations, change is an essential and ongoing process which, if carried out successfully, allows them to evolve and improve their products and services in order to meet the demands of consumers and be competitive. The arguments for and against any changes in health services are hotly debated from local ward to parliamentary level, in local and national press and in the pages of health and medical journals.

The NHS is highly politicized and the appearance of it being strategically and operationally managed by the government of the day remains a strong criticism. A *British Medical Journal* editorial suggests that the NHS is 'unusual in not having a leader' and claims that 'if there is a leader then it is the Secretary of State for Health' (Smith, 2003a). Reasons for this view are proposed by Walshe (2003: 108) who argues that since the NHS's inception, the Secretary of State for Health has been held accountable to Parliament 'for every dropped bedpan, trolley wait, cancelled operation or long waiting list'. The lines of accountability and responsibility, described by Walshe as a 'managerial nonsense but a political reality', have caused an increasing need to centralize and manage every detail creating an ever tightening cycle of control and accountability through a 'hyper-interventionist style of micromanagement' (2003: 108). Political pressure for change comes from the need for successive governments and Health Ministers to stamp their personal authority, usually by imposing structural changes, which give the appearance of important, strategic and instant change (Walshe, 2003).

The change agenda

The long history of change, the scope of policy implementations, the extent of their ramifications, and the ongoing effects on patients and staff within the health services, particularly in England and Wales, are almost overwhelming. There can be few governmental responsibilities to have endured such constant change at the hands of politicians as healthcare. Yet, at the same time, the service is berated, by the same politicians, for not changing sufficiently and requiring further and deeper reform. The Director of Policy at the King's Fund notes the pressure and dilemmas of the government's role:

> On the one hand it has been responsible for the huge central drive and investment to modernise the service. NHS staff are groaning from the number of policies they are required to implement. On the other hand, the pace of change has not been nearly fast enough to satisfy politicians, who demand nothing less than a 'step change' or transformation in the quality of patients' experience. Deep frustration has set in, and awkward questions are now asked at the highest level as to how best to improve performance in a large state-bureaucracy. (Dixon, 2002: 1900)

Walby et al. (1994: 1) further argue that health work has been at the cutting edge of a 'politically inspired attempt to restructure working practices in Britain over the last decade' and that this has turned the health service into a 'laboratory of experimentation in changing work practices'. More recently, Goodlee (2006) bemoans the relentless change, aligning the NHS to a political football and expresses her concern at the waste of energy and goodwill of staff and patients affected by continual policy change. Yet the imperative for an organization to survive depends on its ability to harness and master the process of change.

In 2002, in making the case for public service reform, the then Prime Minister agreed that the creation of the Health Service was a huge achievement and appropriate at a time of post-war austerity but admited that it is 'a product of that age' and 'it no longer meets the needs and challenges in an age of growing prosperity and consumer demand' (Blair, 2002: 1, 3).

On the whole, for the first 25 years of its existence, the NHS was relatively stable. However, post-1974, reforms occurred with increasing speed and have culminated in virtually constant change since 1997 (Davies and Harrison, 2003; Greener, 2004). Walshe (2003) suggests that there has been some kind of organizational upheaval somewhere in the NHS almost every year for the last 20 years and that the pace of change is increasing.

Besides the 1974 reorganization when the service's flawed 1948 structure, problems of duplication and lack of co-ordination were finally recognized (Baggott, 2004), Harrison and Lim (2003) identify two other watershed reorganizations in its history: the 1984 implementation of 'general management' (DHSS, 1983) and the 1991 introduction of the 'internal market' (DH, 1989) – all derived from Conservative government initiatives.

The change cycle

In August 1972, in the White Paper which was the precursor to the 1974 reorganization in England, the Conservative Secretary of State for Social Services (Keith Joseph), stated that while respecting the 'massive performance' and achievements of the NHS, he had come to recognize 'that while this good work will continue, nothing like its full potential can be realised without changes in the administrative organization of the service' (DHSS, 1972a: v).

Twenty-five years later, and after many subsequent 'reforms', writing in the Preface to *The New NHS, Modern, Dependable* the Prime Minister reflected the same opinion:

As we approach the fiftieth anniversary of the NHS, it is time to reflect on the huge achievements of the NHS. But in a changing world no organization, however great, can stand still. The NHS needs to modernise in order to meet the demands of today's public. (DH, 1997: 3)

This watershed document was the first opportunity a Labour government had of reorganizing (variously described as 'reforming', 'modernizing', 'renewing', 'redesigning') the NHS for 18 years and was presented to the country within eight months of coming to power. It further states:

But we also have to change the way that the NHS itself is run. The introduction of the internal market by the previous Government prevented the health service from properly focusing on the needs of patients. It wasted resources administering competition between hospitals. This White Paper sets out how the internal market will be replaced by a system we have called 'integrated care', based on partnership and driven by performance. It forms the basis for a ten year programme to renew and improve the NHS through evolutionary change rather than organizational upheaval. (DH, 1997: 4–5)

The ideas of 'integration', 'partnership', 'performance' and 'evolutionary change', key concepts in managing change in public sector services, are raised here as if new. However, in 1972, Keith Joseph made similar claims. In justifying the move away from a tripartite system, he declared he needed to:

Concentrate instead on ensuring that the two parallel authorities – one local, one health ... shall work together in partnership for the health and social care of the population. This White Paper demonstrates the Government's concern to see that arrangements are evolved under which a more coherent and smoothly interlocking range of services will develop for all the needs of the population. The aim would be to set objectives and standards and to measure performance against them. A sound management system would be created at all levels. (DHSS, 1972a: vi–vii)

The language of 1972 may be less 'modern' than 1997 but the aims and values are similar: good public sector management, efficiency, integrated quality care and cost effectiveness. This has led to criticisms that the process of reform is circular and the different administrations merely recycle and rename the same ideas (Walshe, 2003). Two and a half years after the 1997 White Paper, *The NHS Plan* (DH, 2000a: 2), promoted as a 10-year plan for reform with over 360 targets, again states that 'despite its many achievements, the NHS has failed to keep pace with changes in our society'. Moreover, in the Prime Minister's introduction, he claims that 'Its systems of working are often unchanged from the time it was founded, when in the meantime virtually every other service we can think of has changed fundamentally' (DH, 2000a: 8).

The focus on staff

The leverage used in the *NHS Plan* is the rhetorical device of '1948' whereby its founding principles and values are celebrated as good and constant yet its actions and the actions of its staff are dismissed as 'a 1940's system operating in a 21st century world':

Staff in the health service have tried to lead change. In many places they are doing just that. Their efforts to modernize services all too often founder on the fault lines in the NHS which are a hangover from the world of 1948. (DH, 2000a: 26)

This motif was similarly employed by the NHS Modernization Board's annual report for 2000/2001 stating:

Perhaps the greatest challenge is to achieve the cultural change needed to be able to meet patients' expectations. This requires a fundamental rethink of the way we work together throughout the service to really deliver what people want. In this way the success of *The NHS Plan* rests quite literally on the people working in the NHS and social services. To meet the vision outlined in *The NHS Plan*, we will all have to embrace change on a massive scale. This means no less than a fundamental shift in our working practices and attitudes, some of which have remained unchanged since 1948. (NHS Modernisation Board, 2002: 5)

This is repeated in *Delivering the NHS Plan* (DH, 2002a: 3) when the model's ability to meet twenty-first century health needs is discredited. The outdated system of a 'monolithic top down centralized NHS' must be replaced with a 'devolved health service'.

One of the main differences between the changes foreseen in 1972 and those in 2000 was the message to health service staff and the different values placed on them. Joseph put his faith in the professional status and knowledge of practitioners and was clear that their roles would remain essentially unchanged.

The organizational changes will not affect the professional relationship between individual patients and individual professional workers on which the complex of health services is so largely built. [They] ... will retain their clinical freedom – governed as it is by the bounds of professional knowledge and ethics and by the resources that are available – to do as they think best for their patients. This freedom is cherished by the professions and accepted by the government. (DHSS, 1972a: vii)

This contrasts with a section entitled 'working differently' in *Shifting the Balance of Power* (DH, 2001a). Apart from 'empowering patients' three key aspects are emphasized for long term reform:

(i)   breaking down demarcation between different professional groups and organizations;
(ii) freeing 'frontline' staff to redesign services;
(iii) involving patients in planning their care.

Behind these aspirations were the twin aims of creating cultural and structural change and claims that 'working differently' means:

Giving front-line staff and patients the opportunity to think and work differently to solve old problems in new ways is the only way to deliver the improvements set out in the *NHS Plan*. The changes ... will provide a structure that supports the devolution of power to frontline staff and patients. However a change in culture and new ways of working within organizations will be needed if we are to improve the quality of the patients' experience. (DH, 2001a: 23)

However, the report *Making a Difference* casts doubt on both the effectiveness of the context of care to support these ideas and health professionals themselves who could be more effective in managing and implementing change:

The context of care is changing but nurses, midwives and health visitors are often constrained by structures that limit development and innovation. The NHS and wider health arena needs a modern and responsive workforce of well-motivated, well-trained professionals equipped to respond to the challenges of change. (DH, 1999: 13)

The *NHS Plan*, described by Bradshaw (2002: 1) as a 'massively detailed mega strategy' suggests how this re-invigorated workforce would work:

> NHS staff, at every level, are the key to reform … to deliver the major improvements in patient services the country needs. Radical changes are needed in the way staff work to reduce waiting times and deliver modern, patient-centred services. This is not a question of staff working harder. It is about working smarter to make maximum use of the talents of all the NHS workforce … Managers and clinicians across the NHS must make change happen. (DH, 2000a: 82)

The supporting websites were more bullish. Under one of the 10 key priorities entitled 'Workforce' the target was defined as 'recruiting more staff to the NHS, enhancing their skills, and giving them the incentives and freedom to work in new, more flexible ways'. Staff across the health and social services are the linchpin of change – they will need to:

- work in new, more flexible ways;
- develop and demonstrate leadership;
- play a full part in re-engineering services around the needs of patients (DH, undated a).

Achieving the key priority 'Faster and easier access to services' (DH, undated b), means 'redesigning services and working in new ways so treatment is more convenient for the patient'.
Achieving the key priority 'Quality' means:

- Giving patients comprehensive information about how NHS organizations are performing;
- Regularly asking patients for their views and acting on them (DH, undated c).

In 2004, the *NHS Improvement Plan* (DH, 2004a: 5) claimed that 'frontline staff are being incentivised to become increasingly innovative and creative'. Under a heading 'More staff working differently', it states that there is

> a significant appetite for developing new roles in the service. Attitudes to workforce flexibility have also changed … in addition to their extended clinical roles nurses will be given a lead role in improving the experience of patients in both the hospital and the community. (2004a: 59)

In 2005, the plans for a 'patient-led NHS' argue that still not enough is being achieved. The Chief Executive of the NHS states:

> But the ambition for the next few years is to deliver a change which is even more profound – to change the whole system so that there is more choice, more personalised care, real empowerment of people to improve their health – a fundamental change in our relationships with patients and the public. In other words, to move from a service

that does things *to* and *for* its patients to one which is patient-led, where the service works *with* patients to support them. (DH, 2005: 3)

The means of achieving this objective is through changing culture and systems, giving more authority and autonomy to staff, tackling the barriers which create rigidity and creating new models of change. Within the new 'innovative' NHS, there will be a 'new type of professional' with 'scope for more creativity' and this will involve 'freeing up the entrepreneurialism ... and developing new types of provider organizations' (DH, 2005: 15).

It is with this background that health professionals are expected to implement a wide range of policy directives, develop new services, work in 'new, more flexible ways' and 're-engineer' services. They are encouraged and expected to embrace post-Fordist principles through being flexible, empowered and self-regulating whilst working in one of the most bureaucratized and centrally controlled institutions of the modern age (Klein, 1999; Bradshaw, 2002).

The challenge of change

Implementing change in healthcare is difficult, challenging and often results are short-lived (Parkin, 1997). The delivery of healthcare operates in complex systems where collections of individuals act in unpredictable and diverse ways, where tensions and paradoxes are created through opposing forces of competition and co-operation and where decisions and actions about care are dominated by the unique contexts, priorities and choices facing practitioners (Plsek and Greenhalgh, 2001). For example in mental health, Hall (2006) suggests that nurses' basic assumptions often focus on how difficult their role is and their lack of control or success in managing any change. These assumptions are embedded in their culture leading to poor patient and professional experience and, more worryingly, ambivalence towards implementing change.

The perpetual cycles of imposed change can therefore engender deeply cynical and dismissive attitudes by staff with reactions of 'we've seen it all before, nothing works, just ignore it and keep your head down as it won't last' (Walshe, 2003: 108). Concerns arise about whether devolution of power to frontline staff can actually happen in a system which is 'highly politicized, media sensitive and government-controlled' (Ferlie and Shortell, 2001: 300). Within the 'machine bureaucracy' of the health service, tighter controls mean fewer opportunities for local innovation; reducing opportunities for innovation will reduce variations in service provision; reducing variations means that comprehensive, adaptable and locally appropriate responses to clients' needs will be less likely and the aims of the plan will never be achieved.

It is these arguments that provide the underpinning motivation and rationale for this text. Its central concern is to enable health professionals and equip them with knowledge appropriate for the confident implementation of sound and worthwhile changes in the complex arena of their workplaces.

Table 1.1   Potential change initiatives for healthcare practitioners

- Quality assurance issues
- Clinical effectiveness and standards
- Cost effectiveness and waste reduction
- Client/patient participation and satisfaction
- Team effectiveness
- Service development
- Work content
- Target achievement
- Research implementation
- Management/caseload/workload audit
- Health promoting initiatives
- Continuing Professional Development (CPD)

Aim of the book

The book aims to provide a wide-ranging but practical text for 'frontline' health professionals whose work entails implementing change in its fullest sense; this may mean anything from developing a new multi-disciplinary service for the local community to introducing a journal club within a work team or an evidence-based procedure to a clinical team to improve the quality of care (Table 1.1).

Furthermore the *NHS Plan* requires 'nurses, midwives and therapists to undertake a wider range of clinical tasks including the right to make and receive referrals, admit and discharge patients, order investigations and diagnostic tests, run clinics and prescribe drugs' (DH, 2000a: 83). These examples are simple to state but difficult to achieve. Implementing such change requires the creation of an environment where innovation can take place. Plsek and Wilson (2001) claim that this can be achieved through focusing on four key areas – direction pointing, managing boundaries, gaining permission and managing resources. The challenge is to find ways to gain mastery over these within the traditional roles and specialisms which dominate current healthcare organization and service delivery.

This book, therefore, is about management within healthcare but particularly managing change, since this is essential in any reform programme and yet a significant challenge to staff with little power and authority in the workplace (Bolton, 2004). It aims to reflect the main elements of a project from problem identification and plan development to execution and evaluation. In so doing it provides a compendium of concepts, models, strategies and research which underpins the skills and understanding for managing change in a variety of health environments. It shies away from being a '"how to" recipe that prescribes a number of sequential stages (n-step manuals)' (Dawson, 2003: 3), recognizing the inadequacy of planned change approaches in complex organizations (Plsek and Greenhalgh, 2001; Rhydderch et al., 2004). Though each change project is unique, they share and deal with similar generic features such as political and power environments, territorial and cultural issues, setting aims, outcomes and resources, and these must be assessed and managed through a case by case approach.

Action research

The text integrates management with action research as the core strategy for implementing change in healthcare and this is a key difference from other comparable texts. Explanations of action research are generally found within research texts (Grbich, 1999), but there are few 'management' texts that promote it as a core strategy; indeed it has been claimed that the term is rarely used in management and organizational change literature (Badger, 2000). Yet action research is defined as a management and leadership tool for implementing social change in practical ways and in real situations. Reason (2001) claims that through research, education and socio-political action, action research achieves outcomes which are directly useful to specific groups. Through consciousness raising, reflection and collective self enquiry it empowers groups to develop knowledge and solve problems within their own organization or community thereby promoting organizational learning.

Coughlan and Coghlan unequivocally link action research to the practice of strategic management:

> [Action research] is fundamentally about change. [It] is applicable to the understanding, planning and implementation of change in business firms and other organizations. As action research is fundamentally about change, knowledge of and skill in the dynamics of organizational change are necessary. Such knowledge informs how a large system recognizes the need for change, articulates a desired outcome from the change and actively plans and implements how to achieve that desired future. (2002: 225)

Hall (2006) argues that action research may be more fruitful than traditional models of change as the responsibility for it lies with teams in their workplaces rather than with centralized policy-makers who may be far removed from the situation where change is needed.

MacFarlane et al. (2002) suggest that case studies provide valuable ways of sharing and learning amongst practitioners, particularly for Continuous Professional Development (CPD). Subsequent chapters are illustrated using two thematic action research studies, drawn from national or international health contexts, which demonstrate the relevance of action research to implementing change in healthcare. The generic term 'action research' is used throughout while recognizing that the terms 'participatory action research' (PAR), 'action learning' and 'community development' (CD) are frequently used in the literature (Macaulay et al., 1999). Normally PAR refers to the development of knowledge leading to social action; CD refers to the development of a 'functioning collective' or 'association of citizens' (Lindsey et al., 1999: 1238). Strong links with action research are clear.

The book aims to be of practical use to health professionals who are charged to implement change. The proposed model of change (see Chapter 6) needs a process to drive it and the philosophy and methods of action research, which enable the involvement and participation of practitioners, provides this. As well as meeting the needs of evidence-based practice, action research promotes a philosophy relevant to democratic methods of managing people at work.

Structure of the book

Chapter 2 discusses action research in more detail. It is increasingly recognized as a significant method available to practitioners and is now used frequently in the health and social care arena. It can be used in specific areas with groups of people needing to achieve a solution to a particular problem. Brown and Jones claim that it

> is premised on the assumption that human beings can become knowledgeable about their own situation … therefore [it] is a collaborative venture, where practitioner-researchers work together to achieve three things: first, a better understanding of themselves; second, a better understanding of their situation; and third, overall changes to a situation. (2001: 99)

Hart and Bond discuss a change management project to improve the standards of care in a hospital in the UK which illustrates the importance and relevance of this philosophy:

> Why was it that those involved in commissioning the research selected action research as a strategy to manage change, and what did it offer that other approaches did not? Conversations with key people … suggested that long experience of the National Health Service had convinced them that change imposed from above would be subverted by staff at grass roots level. Action research, with its 'bottom-up' philosophy, seemed to promise a means of overcoming such resistance by promoting a sense of ownership and involvement in those most directly affected by the change. Thus the regional health authority took an enlightened position with regard to the choice of approach. (1995: 90)

This chapter defines and discusses key aspects of action research locating it within the post-modern era as a contrast to the traditional methods of 'positivism'. It outlines key features of the process particularly relating it to the management of change in organizations. It tracks its historical roots, outlines its advantages, disadvantages and methods and considers the debates over rigour, validity, reliability and ethics.

Chapter 3 discusses the social, cultural and organizational contexts of change in society and their influences on healthcare. It outlines the effects of globalization and new communications and information technology, as well as the growing significance of health consciousness and information in creating a more demanding consumer group and the effect of this on health professionals' expertise.

From global issues, it moves onto local, social and organizational contexts of change. It analyses Fordism, post-Fordism and post-modernism and their influence on the organization of public service work. It tracks the rise of the supermarket approach to healthcare, increasing patient knowledge and expectations and the creation of a patient-led NHS (DH, 2005) linking these to the wider changes in society.

Chapter 4 examines management and managing in healthcare and outlines managerial roles and functions. It briefly analyses two managerial approaches commonly applied in healthcare contexts, and contrasts approaches of 'general managers' with those of health professionals from medicine and nursing. Building on Chapter 3, it contrasts modern flexible management with Taylorist/scientific approaches frequently seen within the sphere of nursing.

It concludes with an updated version of a model of management (Figure 4.1) (Parkin, 1998) highlighting key aspects of the management process.

Chapter 5 looks at the controversial place of leadership in the NHS. There are many debates about leadership and both researchers and practitioners appear far from understanding its meaning and complexities in the public sector. It is one of the features of dynamic language that words become fashionable and develop a cachet (Appleyard, 2005). Many recent health policy documents appear to prefer the term 'leadership' to 'management'. For example, under the heading 'Leadership' the *NHS Plan* states that hospitals should have 'a strong clinical leader … [who] … will be given authority to resolve clinical issues, such as discharge delays, problems such as poor cleanliness … [and] draw up local clinical and referral protocols' (DH, 2000a: 86). Whether these actions should be termed leadership, management or administration is debateable and an aim of this chapter is to question the extent of opportunities for leadership within large bureaucratic healthcare organizations. It discusses approaches to leadership, transformational and transactional leadership and the challenges of leadership within bureaucracies.

Chapter 6 forms the central thrust of the text. Views of change (and hence its success) generally hinge on seeing change as either a planned, episodic and discontinuous event or as a perpetually evolving, developmental cycle with no terminal point. Change models normally reflect these different views. The proposed model of change (Figure 6.4) has been developed from the management model in Chapter 4. This model of change attempts, through its process approach, to see change neither as 'episodic' nor as continuous but as an integration of the two where practitioners have to implement change (with an end point – therefore discontinuous) within an environment where change is characterized by 'the ongoing variations which emerge, frequently, even imperceptibly in the slippages and improvisations of everyday activity' (Orlikowski, 1996: 88–9). The model raises other significant factors that influence implementation success. These critical factors guide further analysis.

Chapter 7 explores the influence of culture in the workplace. Understanding organizational and professional culture is at the heart of managing change in healthcare. It has been claimed that in the public sector there is no room for the innovator (Oldcorn, 1996) and this can apply to the bureaucratic tendencies found within many healthcare organizations. The NHS is a multi-cultural society and each different professional group and specialty has its own image and identity, subcultures, roles and rules of behaviour. These professional cultures are transferred to succeeding generations and perpetuated through socialization processes of education, training systems, teachers, mentors and assessors and through occupational histories and stories.

Bauman (1990) has claimed that for the sake of coherence and identity, groups must postulate an enemy to draw and guard their boundaries in order to secure loyalty and co-operation. This view may help to explain the ongoing conflict between doctors, managers and politicians played out in the pages of medical journals. Implementing change in any area of healthcare creates a potential cultural clash between the various organizational and occupational value systems (Drife and Johnson, 1995) and these forces need to be understood and managed. This chapter develops these ideas through the context of current health policies. It considers how culture develops, the meanings and effects of organizational culture, and the different professional cultures within healthcare, examining the challenges for managers and practitioners when initiating change across different professional groups.

Chapter 8 draws on and explores the use of analytical tools. Organizational analysis is often the missing link in change plans as managers are so convinced by their ideas that they do not consider they may be wrong (Harvey-Jones, 1990). This chapter considers organizational learning, examines conditions for its development and proposes methods for analysing and assessing the environment of change. It further explores action research philosophy and its relevance to organizational development (Eden and Huxham, 1996). It proposes a series of questions to ask when planning change (Parkin, 1997) as a means of assessing the organizational climate which is so vital when analysing change opportunities.

Chapter 9 recognizes that resistance to change is an important and natural reaction to change. It defines resistance and examines the roots, forms and characteristics of resistors and resistant organizations. It proposes a range of models of intervention to manage resistance to change.

Chapter 10 proposes that conflict is essential to the growth, change and improvement of organizations. Without conflict, organizations would stagnate. This chapter suggests a positive perspective towards conflict which is often interpreted as a failure in interpersonal relations or organizational systems. It examines the nature and meaning of conflict in healthcare and proposes strategies for its management.

Chapter 11 brings the preceding chapters together to examine strategies for implementing change. It discusses key interpersonal processes and roles from the management model in Figure 4.1 and stresses the importance of self-awareness and flexibility in implementation style. It examines a range of people-based interventions and builds on the attributes of the learning organization – with person- and team-centred management and participation as key strategies for success.

Chapter 12 provides concluding comments on the main issues surrounding managing change in healthcare. It is intended that the book will act as a compendium but with a strongly articulated and realistic statement of caution. Despite a sound idea, the best intentions and the highest motivation, there are innumerable obstacles to disrupt and prevent progress. There are few situations in healthcare which have a high degree of certainty and health professionals need to cultivate a flexible approach to change implementation.

Integrating chapter themes and action research studies

The text aims to integrate action research studies from a range of health and social care fields with implementing and managing change. Major databases including Academic Search Premier, Blackwell Synergy, CINAHL, Emerald and Sage were searched using the key words 'action research' linked with each chapter's theme (e.g.: 'manage*', 'leader*', 'change', 'culture', 'conflict').

Regarding currency, although action research has a longer history in healthcare, databases were searched from 1995, recognizing Hart and Bond's (1995) publication as a significant trigger in raising awareness of action research in health and social care.

This search method produced copious material. Most studies however, though often service wide in scope, originate from a 'nursing' perspective and academic nursing journals. Searching the *British Medical Journal* for example, captured only a handful of genuine action research studies. Furthermore, many citations were limited to analyses of methodology (such as rigour, ethics, validity) or the challenges of action research processes rather than following the convention for research publications of context, method and outcome. This may be a case of 'fighting the corner' for action research and dealing with the enduring methodological criticisms.

To qualify as exemplars, the inclusion criteria are that studies should:

- report a real issue of change management and research significance
- be triggered by a clear and definite problem geared to service improvement
- relate directly to the chapter theme
- involve a group/organization process rather than an individual reflection
- report details of the recursive process of planning, action, reflection and re-planning (see Figure 2.1) rather than single methodological issues.

Following Grbich's (1999) classification, cited studies generally follow an 'organizational' or 'professionalizing' focus where researchers and practitioners work in collaboration to improve practice rather than exploring 'experimental' or 'empowering' approaches.

Livesey and Challender (2002) make two useful points in assessing action research studies. Firstly, they acknowledge that the absence of a declared methodology limits the reader's ability to appreciate the process used to obtain results. Secondly, all studies face the impossibility of capturing the many deep complexities involved in the action world. The boxed examples are further précis to illustrate and emphasize chapter content and readers are encouraged to access the original papers. Finally, there are many terms available to identify the groups to whom this book is aimed. Though it promotes action research as a method of implementing change, frontline staff may not see themselves as 'action researchers'; though they may have a management role, they may not see themselves as 'managers'; and though they wish to make changes, they may not welcome the somewhat pretentious label 'change agent'. The term used throughout the text is 'health professional' as this is inclusive, accurate and the term preferred by NICE (2005).

2

Action Research as a Strategy for Implementing Change

Introduction

In a robust attack on traditional research approaches Greenwood states:

> People do two things: they make observations ... and they perform actions. The most important difference between making observations and performing actions is the intention with which they are done ... in making observations the intention is to discover what is the case, i.e. it is *theoretical* ... In performing actions, however, the intention is to bring about change, i.e. it is *practical*. (Greenwood, 1984: 79–80)

Greenwood asserts that since healthcare is a practical discipline and a social phenomenon that refers to people, their behaviour and interactions, and to groups and institutions and their interrelationships, then action research is a more appropriate research strategy. Practice, she argues, is specific and local, full of concrete content but inherently dynamic. Discussing change in healthcare management generally and organizational development in particular, Bate (2000: 480) claims that action research has been 'inseparable' from change management and specifically it is useful in relation to 'learning' or 'knowledge-creating' organizations (see Chapter 8). Thomas et al. (2005) develop this by maintaining that there is now a growing recognition that models developed from learning organizations and action research are effective in managing change in healthcare.

This chapter discusses action research as a method of implementing change and:

- contrasts its philosophy with traditional research;
- outlines its historical roots;
- sets out its methods and potential weaknesses.

Traditional research

The clinical practice of medicine and other health related occupations is based on universal knowledge created through the 'modernist' tenets of the rational scientific approach. Practice is based on the assumption that in the real world there are patterns, causes and consequences that are natural, regular and enduring and, hence, predictable. Hodgkin (1996) claims that two 'modernist' beliefs form the basis of clinical trials and most medical practice: first, the enduring belief that there is one truth 'out there' which can be known, understood and controlled by those who are rational and competent; and, secondly that there exists the potential to achieve objective understanding of reality which is true for all times and places. As Chalmers observes:

> Science is to be based on what we see, hear, and touch rather than on personal opinions or speculative imaginings. If observation of the world is carried out in a careful, unprejudiced way then the facts established in this way will constitute a secure, objective basis for science. (Chalmers, 1999: 1)

Principles of positivism are based on a belief in objective reality: knowledge gained from empirical data, isolated from its context, validated by independent observers yielding phenomena which can be subjected to empirical testing. Alderson (1998) maintains that medicine is based on its use of reliable, hard data with emphasis on diagnoses and treatments and assumes that these are universally constant, replicable facts.

Outcomes of positivist science are claimed to be context free, value-neutral, validated by logic and measurement, have the consistency of prediction and control and carried out by researchers who are detached from their subjects (Alderson, 1998; O'Brien, 1998; Coughlan and Coghlan, 2002), thus, evidence-based medical practice, and the gold standard of clinical trials, promise certainty (Hodgkin, 1996). As May (2001: 10) concludes, 'the results of research using this method of investigation are then said to be "true", precise and wide-ranging "laws" of human nature'.

Doctrines of modernity

Berge (2001) claims that believing in scientific rationality and secularization was inspirational in ushering in the epoch of modernity as a protest against the traditions of folk and religious beliefs from earlier centuries. Howe (1994) identifies *pre-modern* Europe as seeing the world as pre-ordained, managed and controlled by God through his divine order. Truth was to be revealed by God and uncritically accepted by humankind through his Word. Knowledge was transmitted through narratives – story telling – which reinforced social conventions and, through the power of the storyteller, controlled and promoted social unity (Seidman, 1994).

In contrast, *modernity* arose within a distinct set of intellectual, historical and social circumstances in Western Europe. These developments include the scientific revolution in the sixteenth and seventeenth centuries and the Enlightenment Project and Industrial Revolution in the eighteenth century.

The emergence of science coincided with a decline in religious belief. It offered the opportunity for alternative explanations of the world and enabled people to discover, examine, understand and control it. Discoveries in physics, astronomy and biology challenged the previous traditional religious authority which was dismissed as ignorance, superstition and a sign of an inferior civilization (Seidman, 1994). The creation of scientific measurement and instrumentation allowed increasingly detailed examination of nature to uncover 'objective' truth – the telescope to observe stars and the microscope (the symbol of positivist objective examination, Alderson, 1998: 1007) to study cells. Thus began the move towards considering the world and the body as machines independent of an all-powerful deity (Howe, 1994).

The Enlightenment focused on the importance of social structures and laws leading to the dominance of the concepts of justice, liberty, individualism and human rights and a belief in the pre-eminence of human progress. Knowledge began to be classified into distinct bodies such as psychology and biology. The development of medicine was itself an Enlightenment project, designed to free people from the burden of illness and disease (Dent, 1995).

As Charlton (1993: 497) claimed 'Modernity is a world in a state of progress towards the goal of enlightenment – objective progress through the application of rationality'. Modernism therefore rejected religious thought as the basis of truth and replaced it with rationality, reason and science. As Howe observes, it was Reason which lead to truth, not Revelation:

> Moderns detach themselves from the Universe in order to examine it, probe it, penetrate it, fathom it, see of what it is made, understand how it works, explain it, control it, use it, and exploit it … [They] proceed by *rationally* investigating objects and events in terms of their internal properties, their essential character, nature's universal laws. (Howe, 1994: 514)

The consequence of modernism resulted in the development of so-called meta-narratives such as 'science' (described by Lyotard (1984) as *métarécits*) that competed with and challenged pre-modern religious narratives such as Christianity and Buddhism. O'Mathúna explains that a meta-(grand) narrative transcends time and place and seeks to explain the world from its own particular perspective while attempting to justify its existence: 'Adherents to one meta-narrative believe theirs is the true one, and all the other meta-narratives are wrong. They will try to convince others, using reason, magic, or war, or whatever methods their meta-narrative values' (O'Mathúna, 2004: 4).

The scientific meta-narrative justifies its position through the application of its methods – positivism – generally accepted as involving quantitative measurement, hypothesis testing and causal analysis (Hammersley, 2004). Morrison and Lilford (2001: 437) describe modernism's method as a continually improving and progressive world through rationality and application of the scientific method:

1 Description of what can be observed and an assessment of its patterns.
2 Formulation of an overall theory.

3   Formulation of testable hypotheses.
4   Collection of evidence, under specific and repeatable conditions, leading to the falsification or support of the hypotheses.
5   Examination and proposal of the theoretical and practical implications of the evidence.

Since medicine fully embraces the modernist/scientific approach and is 'modernity in action' it now finds itself in an 'anomalous position ... an island of rationalistic modernity floating in a shifting sea of subjective post-modernity' (Charlton, 1993: 497).

In a similar vein, Rolfe (2006) claims that modernism remains 'undoubtedly the dominant paradigm in nursing at the present time' and that, in healthcare generally, the modernist stance can be seen in the evidence-based medicine movement and the trend towards the randomized clinical trial (RCT) as the highest form of evidence (Rolfe, 2001).

In an analysis of four doctrines of modernity, Walker (2005) suggests that they demand serious consideration of their current relevance to, and impact on, nursing science.

Logocentricity – where the naming of an idea or phenomenon has the effect of reifying or bringing it into existence. This can be seen in the practice of diagnosing and labelling a set of phenomena thereby creating a pre-determined cognitive journey. Its aim is a quest for an authoritative language revealing truth and moral rightness (Seidman, 1994).

Binary logic – where power influences can be applied to situations, decisions or data where 'either/or' can imply 'right or wrong' and particular outcomes can be enforced. Cartesian dualism is an example that promotes one area (the body) over another (the mind). Seidman (1994) adds further binary oppositions as masculine/feminine, nature/culture and cause/effect. He argues that these oppositions lie at the core of Western culture yet do not represent equal values – the first is considered superior, the second, as undesirable and subordinate. Alderson (1998) suggests that modern medicine itself has blurred the edges of such concepts as life and death rendering treatment decisions more complex. In his case against modernism, Walker (2005) argues that 'both/and' promotes inclusiveness compared to 'either/or'.

Privileged voice – where a dominant order, formed through a masculine, Eurocentric history built on establishments such as the Church, medicine and law oppresses and marginalizes weaker groups such as the poor, disabled, older people and other minority categories. Walker (2005) claims this motif has failed and opportunities should be found through research to give voice to marginalized groups in healthcare.

Individualism – where classical liberal theory promotes personal freedom, autonomy and self-determination as a right. This ensures that the locus of decisional control rests within the individual and that personal rights are paramount to and privileged over social obligations. In contrast to this motif, Walker suggests a refocus on human relationships which allows expressions of individualism within groups and communities (Walker, 2005).

Spitzer (1998) argues that the 'modern' project, based on the Newtonian machine paradigm for the last 300 years, is incapable of producing the right configuration for understanding and managing complexity in the modern world (Plsek and Greenhalgh, 2001). As Howe (1994: 530) concludes 'modernity expects knowledge to be consistent and coherent, cumulative and progressive, integrated and unidirectional'.

Post-modernism

In contrast to modernism, post-modernism posits that truth is not 'out there' waiting to be discovered – there are no transcendent criteria of truth (Howe, 1994), no meta-narratives of progress, no centres of authority, no universal systems of beliefs (Lyotard, 1984), no over-arching frameworks to steer by (Hodgkin, 1996). Certainty is replaced by scepticism around what counts as knowledge and who determines validity (Alderson, 1998).

Truth is 'decentred and localised so that many truths are recognized in different times and different places' (Howe, 1994: 520); reality is constructed by people through their language. Truth need not be based on any particular belief system but on an agreed basis within a society or group at a particular time (Raithatha, 1997). Truth is 'not based on reality but on the status of those who are charged with saying what counts as true' (Foucault, 1980: 113). In abandoning absolute standards, post-modern science favours local, contextual and pragmatic strategies (Seidman, 1994). In place of the *métarécits*, post-modernism promotes the *petit récit*, the small narratives from lived lives, which are individual, subjective, diverse, complex and unique (Lyotard, 1984).

Doctrines of post-modernity

Howe (1994) claims that certain aspects, or 'influences', of post-modernity can be recognized in contemporary social work (and by extrapolation, healthcare) theory and practice. These contrast significantly with 'doctrines of modernity' and have noticeable similarities with the philosophy underpinning action research.

Pluralism – this recognizes difference, multiplicity, diversity, the loss of belief in universal explanations of the world. It sees the world as unstable and unpredictable; knowledge is tentative and incomplete and therefore there exist many truths of equal validity. Furthermore, if there are no universal truths then 'differences' should not only be toler-ated but celebrated as a reflection of the 'non-consensual' nature of the social world. No group has a monopoly on the truth or control over what is valued, nor should any group define the experience of another – what is 'natural' in one area may be 'un-natural' in another (Howe, 1994).

Participation – this demonstrates the development of relevance and meaning. If there are no 'privileged perspectives' or 'absolute authorities' (which are modernist constructs), then truths are working and relative; practical judgements are formulated through the full participation of all those involved in decisions. Meaning is developed in the context in which people find themselves and in collaboration with others; as meaning develops *in situ*, so this legitimizes actions.

Power – Howe (1994) argues that post-modern analyses no longer accept that the knowledge base of social workers is determined by the nature of the diagnosed condition – rather it is mediated through local and situational access to professional and specialist knowledge and skill; as all-encompassing theories of society and history (meta-narratives) are undermined, they become less certain, less reliable and therefore lose their power. As Lyotard explains (1984: xxiv) 'I define postmodern as incredulity toward meta-narratives'.

Many observers argue that post-modernism is a highly contested construct and should not be simplified to the extent that it is regarded as a complete relaxation of the rules and methods of science (Rolfe, 2006). Others reject its relevance entirely (Kermode and Brown, 1996).

In his analysis of its contested state, Rolfe makes a distinction between those who adopt an extreme relativist position, where there is no reality 'out there', but claim reality is constructed separately by each individual, and that truth is 'subjective, multiple and fractured' (Rolfe, 2006: 9). These, he calls 'judgemental relativists'. Alternatively, those who adopt a more questioning stance towards taken-for-granted assumptions about truth and its origins he classifies as 'post-modern ironists'. Rolfe claims that 'post-modern ironists' would argue that the idea of a scientific and single 'gold standard' for judging truth makes no sense:

> How is it, for example, that the RCT is taken as the 'gold standard' for healthcare research rather than, say, the phenomenological interview, the ethnographic participant observation, or even the introspective reflection of the healthcare practitioner? The modernists would claim that the RCT provides better or more accurate information on which to base healthcare decisions, whereas the post-modernists would point out that, in a decentred universe, there are no absolute standards against which to measure those claims … the post-modernists point out that there are no good reasons why we *should* judge research methods against the modernist scientific criteria of the RCT. (Rolfe, 2001: 41)

Post-modernists therefore propose that the absolutism of modernism is no longer an acceptable or appropriate way of understanding the world (Brown and Jones, 2001). To summarize: in the pre-modern age truth was found through God and his word; from the pre-modern to the modern, God was replaced by the scientific instrument and what it revealed; from the modern to the post-modern, the instrument is replaced by the individual and what she or he thinks and feels.

Action research

Action research can claim to share many 'post-modern' aspects in its underpinning principles since its methods go beyond the confines of the scientific paradigm (Rolfe, 1996). Hart and

Bond (1995: 21) claim that modern day action researchers 'do not seek to find universal laws of human behaviour through which behaviour can be measured' rather they emphasize awareness raising, empowerment, collaborative working and for practitioners themselves to become action researchers. It operates from a specific value objective to promote democracy and emancipation, recognizing that there is unequal distribution of power and resources in the world (Brown and Jones, 2001). Berge (2001: 281) claims that in the historical era of 'later modernism' action research 'could be a useful method to enhance social justice in local contexts'.

Criticism has been levelled at the 'theory–practice' gap in clinical practice where research results do not always fit the uniqueness of many practice situations in healthcare (Meyer, 2000). Action research, on the other hand, has arisen amid growing criticism of positivism, in particular its applicability to the context in which care is being delivered and its ability to understand the complexities and subtleties of caring for human health and illness (Morrison and Lilford, 2001; Plsek and Greenhalgh, 2001).

Quoss et al. (2000: 51) describe action research as a 'post-modern mode of inquiry' and Grbich (1999: 211) describes a type of 'post-modern action research' which de-emphasizes the search for truth and in contrast looks for ways knowledge is produced, which groups exert power and who benefits. Hence, inherent power structures within and between groups and organizations can be examined and identified in order to restructure and transform them. Order, hierarchy and rationality are rejected in favour of flexibility (see Chapter 3).

The primary purpose of action-based research is to bring about change in specific situations, in local systems and real-world environments with aims to solve real problems. As such it is context-bound, those within the locality participate and collaborate demonstrating major differences with traditional research. Box 2.1 illustrates action research's philosophy of involvement and improvement at the local level.

Box 2.1

Overview

Leighton (2005) reports on a study concerning a 12- and a 6-bedded mental health rehabilitation unit in the UK designed to assist institutionalized patients to normalize within society using a modified therapeutic community approach. However, problems were encountered affecting success – these included inappropriate admissions, lack of suitable placements, user over-dependence and sick-role activity, and financial restrictions leading to 'bed-blocking'. The smaller unit was closed leaving the 12-bedded unit directionless and isolated from the mental health services, running at 60 per cent capacity and closed to student placements.

Exploratory and planning phase

Service users, relatives and unit staff undertook a review and audit of mental health rehabilitation services in the area. A staff focus group was held to identify historical problems and group experience of the unit and a literature review undertaken. Data

---

generated were measured against government and Trust policies. This revealed the unit had suffered from: inconsistent management; erratic funding; inappropriate admissions requiring specialist input; non-rehabilitative care; creation of over-dependence of users; staff suffering low morale; poorly defined rehabilitative pathways from admission to discharge; and lack of facilities for users with combined clinical and social needs.

Decision and action phase

A steering group was created. Managers, staff and users agreed a range of problem-solving goals with the aim of re-establishing social involvement based on the principles of 'community'.

Their goal was to establish new unit aims based on the 'recovery' model and incorporating:

1. appropriate referrals – governed by age limits, mental state, and motivation;
2. contracts based on the Care Programme Approach;
3. genuine rehabilitative therapies;
4. minimization of user over-dependence;
5. staff involved in meaningful rehabilitation tasks to raise morale;
6. unit integration with its locality.

Second observation/reflection phase

The new system was to be evaluated every 6 months via staff questionnaires, focus groups, audits and user assessments, including:

- staff self-reports – measuring the effectiveness of the new configuration and wider interface with the rehabilitation system;
- service users – focusing on admission, assessment improvements and success in onward placements.

Summary

The self-determination qualities of the action research process assisted in breaking the institutionalized deadlock and breathed new life into the old system. As in many management projects some people became more involved than others and some showed indifference.

Since new knowledge is created or expanded to solve specific problems, action research also develops theory. The 'theory generating' aspect of action research characterizes it as research and significantly differentiates it from other change management approaches (Sandars and Waterman, 2005).

These aspects of action research ensure its suitability in many other professional human and practice-based areas such as education (Elliott, 1991), leadership (Williamson, 2005), management (Eden and Huxham, 1996; Coughlan and Coghlan, 2002), occupational therapy (Taylor et al., 2004), primary care (Nichols, 1997), sport (Frisby et al., 2005), and in wider health related settings generally (Meyer, 2000). Action researchers achieve change through planning interventions, by working with people to help influence their environment, or by providing sufficient information to enable them to take responsibility for making changes. Through this, it actively promotes organizational learning (see Chapter 8).

Eden and Huxham (1996) raise cautions arguing that action research is an 'imprecise, uncertain and sometimes unstable activity' when compared with many other research approaches. Greenwood (1984), however, justifies its appropriateness since it is:

- Situational: it is concerned with diagnosing a problem in a specific context and attempting to solve it in that context.
- Collaborative and participatory: its partnership approach ensures that researchers negotiate their plans and interpretations of the situation with other involved individuals.
- Evaluative: its cyclical nature means that modifications and changes are continually monitored within the situation making it flexible and adaptable. This reflects practice that is dynamic.

Action research may therefore accord with Hodgkin's (1996: 1568) comments regarding definitions of 'truth' from a post-modern view. He claims that to the post-modern eye truth is not 'out there' waiting to be revealed but is something which is 'constructed by people, always provisional and contingent on context and power'.

Action research defined

Definitions of action research are varied and there is little agreement (Dickens and Watkins, 1999). Livesey and Challender (2002) state that the literature is too diverse to present a cohesive view, however Hart identifies the main concepts: '[Action research] is problem-focussed, context specific, participative, involves a change intervention geared to improvement and a process based on a continuous interaction between research, action, reflection and evaluation' (1996: 454).

It is evident from the above that action research differs from traditional research outlined earlier. It attempts to bridge the gap between theory, practice and research and between researchers and practitioners. Dickens and Watkins (1999) outline other differences:

- Traditional research is reductionist in its treatment of human phenomena. Action research works holistically in naturally occurring settings.
- Traditional science assumes substantial knowledge about hypothetical relationships. Action researchers may begin with limited knowledge of the specific situation, requiring work with others to observe, reflect, clarify and change the situation.
- Traditional research collects data and culminates at the point of discovery. Action research collects data expressly to guide future plans.

Bellows (cited Zaner, 1968) distinguishes *static* research and *action* research. He designates the former as 'elemental' or 'analytical' and the latter as 'dynamic'. In action research a 'whole solution is sought for a real problem in a living situation which is commonly complex in nature' (Zaner, 1968: 29).

While Hammersley (2004: 174) maintains that much inquiry does indeed arise in the context of a problem and is concerned with resolving that problem, he asks if action research is a form of research or a form of action. He notes that given its 'context-specific' hierarchy and its primary focus to bring about change in practice rather than produce knowledge, calling it 'inquiry-subordinated-to-another-activity,' he cautions that in practice this can generate contradictions.

Historical roots

Grbich (1999) claims that action research was first used around 1900 by a doctor using group participation and co-researcher methods with prostitutes in a community setting in Vienna. Modern action research developed from the progressive and democratic ideas of Kurt Lewin (1890–1947) as a form of 'rational social management'. His seminal paper in 1946 was a response to a plea to improve inter-group relations in communities in Cleveland, Ohio. He cited his earlier work in Connecticut as being 'action research – research which will help the practitioner' (Lewin, 1946: 34), since it was a way of 'generating knowledge about a social system while, at the same time, attempting to change it' (Elden and Chisholm, 1993: 121). Hart and Bond explain that as Professor of Child Psychology at Iowa University Lewin acted as a consultant to the Harwood factory in Virginia (see Chapter 9) to assess the effect of worker participation on productivity. Workers had grievances about piece rates, turnover, low productivity and output restrictions and expressed aggression towards management. Managers wanted to know why change was resisted so strongly and why, following changes, workers were aggressive, output decreased, and absenteeism and staff turnover increased:

> A theory of frustration was developed based on [Lewin's] field theory and his equilibrium theory of change which hypothesised that frustration arose from a conflict between two opposing forces, the driving force corresponding to the goal of reaching the standard rate for the job, and the resisting force corresponding to the difficulty of the job. (Hart and Bond, 1995: 18)

The experiment to solve these problems at the factory created three work groups; one did not participate in the changes, another participated through representatives and a third participated fully in all aspects and took part in discussion with managers. The results showed that the non-participating groups suffered a fall in production and morale, whereas the fully participating group worked effectively and improved its productivity. Lewin concluded that democratic participation was preferable in solving work-group problems to the 'coercion' commonly associated with scientific management (see Chapter 4) (Hart and Bond, 1995).

The 'scientific' debate

Action research therefore developed in opposition to quantitative research and its claims of 'objectivity', reliance on observation and measurement, and tight control over the field of study.

O'Brien (1998) argues that what separates action research from general professional practice, consulting, or daily problem-solving is its emphasis on scientific study. This means that the researcher (or facilitator) manages the problem systematically and ensures that interventions are informed by underpinning theory.

Holter and Schwartz-Barcott (1993) claim that action research does not require any special method of data collection and that models and methods can be both 'explorative and creative'. Furthermore, its philosophy does not preclude the use of traditional data gathering methods (Coughlan and Coghlan, 2002). O'Brien (1998) argues that its holistic approach allows it to employ a variety of methods though these usually reflect a qualitative paradigm (Sandars and Waterman, 2005) yielding 'soft' data and commonly include not only questionnaire surveys, structured and unstructured interviews (such as patient satisfaction surveys), but also journal keeping, document collection and analysis, participant observation, focus groups and case studies (see Box 2.2). 'Hard' data are also important to gather and evaluate, and examples in healthcare may include epidemiological data, treatment inputs, patient throughput and output. Lilford et al. (2003: 103) argue that action research does not preclude the use of any research method and that a study could include a 'series of randomised trials carried out within the iterative cycle'.

Lewin asserts that 'this by no means implies that the research needed is in any respect less scientific or "lower" than would be required for pure science in the field of social events, I am inclined to hold the opposite to be true' (1946: 35). This view is shared by Bate (2000), who claims that action research is not just an evidence-based methodology but rather one of the few examples of an actual process of implementing an evidence-based approach. Coughlan and Coghlan (2002) stress that what is important in action research is that the planning and use of tools is well thought out and clearly integrated in the research process. Furthermore, they claim that action research should 'not be judged by the criteria used in positivistic science, but rather within the criteria of its own terms' (2002: 226).

Eden and Huxham (1996) caution that action research should not be used loosely to cover a variety of approaches, nor as a way of excusing 'sloppy' research, nor as a reason to ignore issues of rigour. Good action research, they stress, should be good science.

In a closely argued paper, Morrison and Lilford (2001) propose three criteria whereby research can be judged as being scientific:

- Explanatory theories are developed.
- Theories are comprehensive in that they apply to the whole domain.
- Theories are falsifiable where persistent test failures count against the theory.

They propose an 'idealized' definition consisting of five 'tenets' found in most action research projects, and promoted by action researchers, which carry an implied criticism of mainstream research. They then judged these against their criteria for a scientific approach:

1 'Flexible planning' – the content and direction are not to be determined at the outset but rather develop as data are collected.
2 'Iterative' – research activity proceeds by a cycle of defining the problem, proposing action, taking action, learning the lessons of that action and reconsidering the problem in the light of those lessons.
3 'Subjective meaning' – the meaning to those involved with the problem should be allowed to determine the content, direction and measure of success of the project.
4 'Simultaneous improvement' – the project must set out to change the situation for the better.
5 'Unique context' – the project must acknowledge the unique nature of the social context.

Though they dispute that action research can be judged as scientific under their stated terms, they do accept that some of its tenets are tailor-made for health services and that they could and should be considered by mainstream researchers, and, if adopted, findings are likely to be more usable by health professionals and managers.

Methods of action research

As yet, no definitive set of guidelines has emerged (Quoss et al., 2000). Coughlan and Coghlan (2002) emphasize that since action research requires dynamic co-operation between the researcher and the client group, the methods require continuous adjustment to new information within a series of unfolding and unpredictable events. As Meyer argues:

> Action research ... relies more heavily on the skills of the enquirer, with the approach being more personal and interpersonal than methodological. As such it is not possible to delineate clearly the stages of action research in advance. Each study is unique and follows its own pattern of development. (Meyer, 1995: 25)

Methods therefore consider the structure, process and outcome triad. However, the dynamism of the situation does not mean that the approach is haphazard. Stringer (1996) suggests a simple format of 'look' (problem definition), 'think' (planning) and 'act' (implementation).

Lewin stresses the importance of planning which is a key function of management operations (see Chapter 4). Planning begins with an examination of a general idea of a problem or issue:

> Planning starts usually with something like a general idea. For one reason or another it seems desirable to reach a certain objective, and how to reach it is frequently not too clear. The first step then is to examine the idea carefully in the light of the means available. Frequently more fact-finding about the situation is required. If this first period of planning

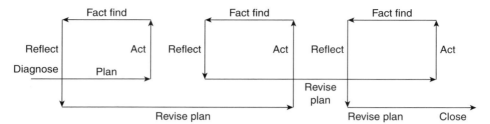

Figure 2.1 The recursive action research cycle

> is successful, two items emerge: namely, an 'over-all plan' of how to reach the objective and secondly, a decision in regard to the first step of action. Usually this planning has also somewhat modified the original idea. The next period is devoted to executing the first step of the original plan. (Lewin, 1946: 37)

This is followed by the collection of baseline data or measurements. Lewin called this 'reconnaissance' or 'fact-finding' which:

1 evaluates the action;
2 gives the planners a chance to learn – to gain new insight;
3 assists in planning the next step;
4 helps to modify the overall plan.

The cycle of fact-finding, planning, action and evaluation is repeated (see Figure 2.1). Each step is assessed determining the next step that may involve modification of the original idea. Lewin continues:

> The next step again is composed of a circle of planning, executing and reconnaissance or fact-finding for the purpose of evaluating the results of the second step, for preparing for the rational basis for planning the third step, and for perhaps modifying again the over-all plan. Rational social management, therefore, proceeds in a spiral of steps each of which is composed of a circle of planning, action and fact-finding about the result of the action. (Lewin, 1946: 38)

These stages are supplemented by actions such as: negotiation, seeking assistance, assessment, investigating, making choices, working through implications, reviewing changes and withdrawing. Lewin claimed that 'fact-finding' was central to action research as it established whether an action led to an improvement. These terms indicate implicitly that action research relates closely with both management and learning:

> If we cannot judge whether an action has led forward or backward, if we have no criteria for evaluating the relation between effort and achievement, there is nothing to prevent us from making the wrong conclusion and to encourage the wrong work habits. Realistic fact-finding and evaluation is a prerequisite for any learning. (Lewin, 1946: 35)

Groups themselves define these issues and instigate, implement and assess action for change in a collaborative manner. In this sense action research is democratic. As Zaner summarizes:

> It must be borne in mind that chief among the purposes of developing a comprehensive plan – essentially an action research plan – is the involvement of the responsible authorities (people) in co-operative planning and subsequently in the implementation of their joint plan or collaborate set of ideas. (Zaner, 1968: 31)

The example in Box 2.2 illustrates these democratic principles at the wider community level.

Box 2.2

Overview

Lindsey and McGuiness (1998) claim that though PAR is gaining in credibility, little is known about how to involve the community in social action. The 'STEPS project', funded by Health Canada's Seniors Independence Program and involving over 166 agencies and organizations, was designed to create a safer environment for those at risk of falling by raising public awareness of falls, reducing hazards and developing 'community hazard reduction risk management plans'.

Exploratory and planning phase

Four qualitative methods were used:

1   *Study-related documents*: committee meeting minutes, media reports, letters of invitation, tape and video news recordings were analysed to assess community involvement.
2   *Participant observation* of STEPS steering group meetings, presentations and member presented workshops.
3   *Individual interviews* with key participants – members of the STEPS steering committee, university researchers, a volunteer and an engineer.
4   *Focus group interviews* with members of the above groups.

All interviews were consented, recorded, transcribed and validated by participants who were purposively sampled from those with significant involvement in the project. Interviews focused on reasons for involvement, experience in the project and views on successful community involvement.

Decision and action phase

The significant elements were summarized under five main themes which emerged from the data.

1   Planning for participation:
    • Develop effective communication strategies.
    • Identify major stakeholders, potential benefits and exchange ideas.

(Continued)

(Continued)

- Identify and invite target groups.
- Identify the political issues and power holders.

2 Structural components of community involvement:
- Develop a steering committee with active, knowledgeable people with broad community interests.
- Facilitate smooth running of committee meetings.
- Involve the community in data collection, analysis and dissemination.
- Timing – PAR projects take considerable time and effort to progress.
- Maintain commitment, recognize achievements, identify barriers and develop strategies to overcome them.
- Wrap up the project – plan a concluding event to provide closure.

3 Living the philosophy of PAR:
- Engage the community in diagnosing the problem and monitoring change.
- Ensure that university and community researchers have congruent values.
- Develop trusting and collaborative partnerships – critical to the success of PAR.
- Promote effective change – the committee anticipated, facilitated and supported effective change.

4 Credibility and the community:
- The reputation of the two university researchers adds credibility.
- The focus of research (safety) addresses the immediate concerns of the community.
- Influential power brokers lend support and promotion to the project.

5 Leadership style:
- PAR is more than employing a set of leadership techniques.
- PAR needs to be guided by a belief in community participation leading to effective change.
- Leadership needs to emphasize facilitation, collaboration, co-ordination, rather than being directive.
- The community should be used as a source of expertise.

Summary

The STEPS project created positive and involving experiences for participants. They experienced personal growth, learning and satisfaction in making a difference to the safety of the community. The results can provide a framework and guidance to others embarking on action research projects.

Building on Lewin's sequence (1946) and Stringer's (1996) look, think and act process, action research phases can be expanded to:

1 **Exploratory/diagnostic/fact finding phase**
- Identification of a problem.
- Fact-finding to develop an overall plan (via work placement observation; staff/patient interviews; SWOT analysis (strengths, weaknesses, opportunities, threats); task analysis; literature reviews).
- Determine measurement tools, if appropriate.

2 **Planning/decision/action phase**
  - May involve modifying the original idea.
  - Considering alternatives.
  - Planning key changes in discussion with participants.
  - Planning strategies of intervention.
  - Taking action.

3 **Evaluation/reflection phase**
  - Critical personal reflection on process, data and learning.
  - Fact-finding (review) of the impact of the action – may be formative or summative.
  - Judgements regarding improvements.
  - Use of group meetings, questionnaires, interviews, reflective diaries.

4 **Second data-collection phase**
  - Repeat of phase 1 concentrating on evaluation of levels of change or achievement.
  - May include focus groups, questionnaires, interviews.
  - Repeat and reflect.
  - Identify lessons learnt.

5 **Evaluation, reflection, re-planning and re-implementation of action**
  - Repetition of cycles 2–4 as necessary.

6 **Final assessment of changes and utilization of results**
  - Closure, theory generation and write-up.

This is not a rigid set of sequences that action researchers must follow religiously, rather researchers should aim to freely flow through the phases (Williamson and Prosser, 2002a) which will vary in time-span depending on the needs, complexity and dynamics of the situation. However, the essential recursive rather than the linear process of traditional research is clear.

Summary of action research

The key aspects of action research can be summarized as being:

- Centred on change and changing workplace situations.
- Problem-focused: solving problems rather than merely collecting data.
- A cyclical process where research, action and evaluation are interlinked.
- Collaborative: based on relationships with participants in the change process.
- Educative: aims at organizational improvement thus promotes organizational learning (see Chapter 8).
- Concerned with individuals as members of social groups.
- Characterized by openness to participants, researchers, methods, change, validity and ethics.
- It creates and develops theory.

Advantages of action research

The principal advantages of action research can be summarized as follows:

- It offers a means of solving local problems.
- It promotes an interest in research amongst those not previously involved.
- It defines individuals as active participants rather than passive subjects.
- Group participation helps motivate and maintain interest.
- Focus of research is usually meaningful to participants.
- Results of change are monitored alongside action for rapid feedback.
- An acceptable and appropriate method for social and healthcare contexts.
- Promotes a 'bottom up' approach to managing change.
- Encourages self-awareness from both participants and researcher.
- Results may be able to inform other, similar, contexts and situations.

Limitations of action research

The main limitations of action research can be summarized as follows:

- Lack of precision over its nature and definition.
- Potential limitations on generalizing findings beyond the local situation.
- Attracts attendant problems of change management including resistance and conflict (see Chapters 9 and 10).
- Can be time consuming for little gain.
- Can encounter cultural, professional and managerial constraints on change initiatives.
- Methods can conflict with notions of autonomy and individualization particularly where they are highly valued.
- Ethical issues require careful explanation and management.

Issues within action research

Ethical issues

The ethical issues within action research delineate it from standard management strategies of change implementation. In most circumstances the vital ethical issues in action research are no different from those in any other research. These include, informed consent for taking part, maintaining confidentiality and accuracy of data, and assurances that participants will not experience harm and have the right to withdraw at any time.

However, given the dynamic and changing nature of data and actions, Williamson and Prosser (2002a) suggest that ethics in action research is more complex and poses particular challenges to researchers. They argue that whereas participants should strive for an ethical stance, there is a need to be aware of the issues, notably the vulnerability of participants. Regarding consent, they ask what are participants consenting to since they cannot know exactly where the journey will lead them. If the research concerns a team, what is the situation if members do not wish to take part, or withdraw from the study midway through – does this compromise their position and are they expected to engage in the final improved state? Other standard research ethics such as confidentiality may pose problems because of the open and collaborative nature of the processes, some data may have to be shared amongst the participants causing discomfort and resentment amongst individuals. When sensitive data are shared with another participant, is the disclosure to a 'co-researcher', 'colleague' or 'friend'? This raises issues of trust, particularly where senior staff or managers are involved in the project. Confidentiality can also be compromised where particular roles can be identified in a report (Williamson and Prosser, 2002b). Williamson and Prosser (2002b) share data from their study into developing the lecturer-practitioner role where Prosser was a participant to Williamson as the researcher. Prosser makes it clear that her consent could not be 'informed' as neither she nor Williamson could know how the study would develop. Furthermore, as there were so few participants, it was likely that she could be identified even though reports were anonymized.

Reliability and validity

Generally action research literature agrees that these concepts, central to the rigour of research, do raise difficult questions. Hope and Waterman (2003) recognize that reliability and validity are derived from positivism and therefore are already value laden, and there is a view that they have no place in action research. They suggest that more alternative terms may be 'ensuring quality' 'credibility', 'transferability' or 'dependability'. Badger (2000) appeals to common sense in that data and arguments are presented in a logical, unbiased, way, but points out that it is more important that researchers are reflexive and aware that their own actions, beliefs and biases can affect research outcomes. This is a strategy used by Marincowitz (2003) who, as researcher and medical practitioner, was open to ideas from other participants through active listening, using reflection in a research diary and being aware of preconceived ideas about mutual participation. Validation of data can be ensured by the facilitator checking with participants either as individuals or within a group, the detail of the analysis and interpretation. This transparency will give first-hand knowledge. As Whyte (1991: 41–2) asserts 'cross checking … provides a higher standard of factual accuracy'. Others have suggested that as the main aim of action research is to change and improve a situation, then the face validity that findings fit reality can be sufficient (Greenwood, 1984) but only tentative generalizations beyond the situation can be made.

Conclusion

Action research is more than simply 'work' and problem solving; it has qualities and constituents above and beyond both 'research' and 'management'. Rather it is a change management approach which uses research methods; in this way it is systematic, scientific, participative and collaborative. Those facilitating action research approaches require deep and critical reflection skills, understanding of both qualitative and quantitative methods and interface management skills, since, to implement change in healthcare it is necessary to cross professional and status boundaries and develop meaningful partnerships. The key way of achieving this is to start from the concerns and problems which participants already own.

Chapter summary

- Action research is a process that focuses on solving local problems, promoting social change and improving the quality of service provision through a democratic process.
- It is participative and educative and involves groups with a common purpose, interest or need.
- Through its philosophy it has been described as a 'post-modern' approach in contrast to traditional approaches.
- It uses progressive and iterative processes of problem identification, planning, action and reflection/analysis.
- Criticisms focus on a lack of definition, the usual difficulties and challenges associated with change (see Chapter 6) and problems with validity and reliability.
- The particular methods used in action research raise issues of a political, ethical and methodical nature that researchers and participants have to manage.

3

The Social Context of Change

Introduction

The world is changing and the pace and extent of change is greater than has previously been experienced. Change is vital for nations and societies, organizations and institutions, families and individuals for their growth, development and survival. If these entities do not change they will lose their place in their particular sphere of influence and be unable to meet their aims and develop their products. Without changing, they will wither and die.

Giddens (1989: 632) states that 'everything changes, all the time' but suggests that to identify significant change means to demonstrate how far and over what period of time there are changes in the *underlying structure* of a situation and, in relation to human groups, what changes are evident in the *basic institutions*. In the above entities it is necessary to continually assess, manage and refine internal and external functions in order to react to events, maintain relationships and develop a competitive edge. These requirements are no different within the sphere of healthcare.

This chapter will outline the significance of wider social changes before focusing on key changes within healthcare. It will then discuss the effects of Fordism, post-Fordism and post-modernism on changes in healthcare, healthcare policies and the work of health professionals.

Current influences on social change

Broadly, the tracking of change is analysed under the headings of political, economic, social and technological developments, however Paton and McCalman (2000) and Scambler (2002) identify several major influences that organizations must be aware of and address in order to successfully manage change. Though these influences are closely connected, they include the following components.

Globalization

Globalization can be defined as interdependent processes through which the peoples of the world are incorporated into a single society (Albrow, 1990). This is evident by the growth in power of the capitalist market place where worldwide business can be dominated by relatively few, large, usually Western, multinational companies and where share values move in concert across financial institutions, stock markets and time zones. The development of instant communication systems promotes worldwide social interaction where breaking news, such as the attack on the World Trade Centre in New York in 2001 can be watched in real time from computers and mobile telephones. The global spread of rapid and efficient supply chains, delivering products from producer to customer, lowers unit costs making products cheaper and more accessible and creating opportunities for greater selection. The growth and monopoly of internet technology such as that provided by Microsoft and Google accelerate the process of shrinking the globe to create a 'one-world' view thereby reducing national cultures and identities. News regarding disease outbreaks such as Severe Acute Respiratory Syndrome (SARS) or Bird Flu in the Far East, can be brought into living rooms in the West and motivate needless preventative health reactions by both individuals and governments in places separated by thousands of miles. These elements remove normal social relations from their local contexts (Scambler, 2002) and hence in healthcare, can cumulatively influence and alter patient and practitioner relationships.

The environment

The growth in worldwide populations together with the expansion of communication systems have been instrumental in raising awareness of pollution, threats to the environment and the limits of the world's raw materials. This has prompted the assessment of the impact of carbon footprints and moves to use alternative, renewable sources of energy. The Carbon Trust reports that 66 per cent of the consumers in the UK surveyed said they wanted to know the carbon footprints of goods they bought and preferred to buy items with low carbon footprints (Osborne, 2006). The 2005 G8 Summit was targeted by worldwide pressure groups to reach agreement regarding Third World debt, economic development in Africa and actions to reduce global warming. The global warming debate has reached a point where attitudes to fossil fuel use, renewable energy and recycling are changing and feeding into alternative developments in policy making in areas such as transport and taxation. Indeed emissions of greenhouse gases in the UK fell by 14 per cent between 1990 and 2002 (Office for National Statistics (ONS), 2006a). Unravelling the mechanisms of such attitudinal changes is a challenge and a necessity for health professionals.

Health consciousness

The increasing incidence of chronic illness is well documented as are continuing health inequalities (Sheaff, 2005). The UK government's response, *Choosing Health* (DH, 2004b), sets out key principles for supporting the public to make healthier, more informed choices. It states that there is growing public awareness of health issues and a greater receptiveness to opportunities to improve health. It claims that health is becoming more prominent in news reports, prompted by the Academy Award Nominee for 'best documentary' in 2004, *Super Size Me*. This film examined the filmmaker's deteriorating health problems from eating only McDonalds for a month to the growing concern of observing doctors. Awareness is also raised by the report *Securing Good Health for the Population* (Wanless, 2004) and the Parliamentary Health Select Committee's report on obesity (House of Commons Health Committee, 2004). This claims that obesity in Britain has grown by almost 400 per cent in the last 25 years and if present trends continue, will surpass smoking as the greatest cause of premature loss of life. Research (Lean et al., 2006) claims that by 2010, a third of all adults in the UK will be classified as obese and that these levels will reduce life expectancy, add to the burden of chronic illness and could bankrupt the health service.

Furthermore, awareness of poor quality food in schools was raised by the 'celebrity' chef Jamie Oliver, who, it is claimed, prompted action by the government within a mere five weeks of his campaign against the poor quality of school food (Blair, 2005). Smoking, and particularly the growing awareness of dangers from passive smoking, led to the smoking ban in all public places in the UK by 2007.

Pressure from a more educated public has prompted greater details on food labelling. Manufacturers are reducing or using alternatives to sugar in soft drinks. The salt content in processed and convenience food is being reduced (Gibson et al., 2000) and there is increased use of omega 3 fatty acids as a protection against cardiovascular disease (Din et al., 2004). A more pluralistic society has prompted a rise in the range of alternative therapies and consultations with therapists (Blane, 1997). This has presented a challenge to orthodox medicine as the legitimate providers of healthcare.

Lifestyle trends

The Statistical Office's annual report on Social Trends (ONS, 2006a) shows radically changing trends in lifestyle, employment and incomes, population, leisure pursuits and education. It shows that the UK is increasingly racially and religiously diverse creating a more pluralistic society and a consequent need to recognize different beliefs, cultures and values to maintain stability (Giddens, 1989). Between 1971 and 2004 those aged under 16 declined by 2.6 million yet those over 65 increased by 2.2 million, prompting concerns about long-term care and pension provision. To counteract these changes the pension age is undergoing a phased increase from 65 to 68 between 2024 and 2046 (The Pension Service, 2008). Marriage break-up has contributed to changes in family structure and increased the number of households by 30 per cent (5.6 million) between 1971 and 2004. Employment trends show that more people are economically active than in the early 1990s. The Labour Force Survey (ONS, 2005) recorded the highest number of people in employment in the UK since it began its records in 1971, though the proportion of the population in work was lower. Furthermore, although there are regional variations, real disposable income has increased by 130 per cent since 1971 and has increased every year since 1982. Higher disposable income has increased car ownership, with two-car households rising from 7 per cent in 1970 to 30 per cent in 2003. Despite an increase in income, however, personal insolvencies increased by 31 per cent from 2003 to 2004 indicating a vast increase in personal debt.

The workplace

Over recent years, government policy has stressed the importance of maintaining a healthy work–life balance. A key factor in this is the increasing flexibility of labour with a growth of 150 per cent in home workers between 1997 and 2006 (ONS, 2006a). Over 20 per cent of full-time and 25 per cent of part-time employees had some form of flexible working arrangement in 2005. The increasing pace of change in job content means more adults attend work-based training schemes but data from employers indicate a skills gap, particularly in communication, customer handling and team-working. Employers report that the main reason for the skills gap was that employees are 'not keeping up with change' (ONS, 2006a: 45). In 1998 the European Commission 'Working Time Directive' was implemented in the UK. The regulations apply to full-time, part-time and temporary workers and provide for an average maximum working week of 48 hours, although individual workers can choose to work longer. Originally doctors in training were excluded but a revision now limits them to 58 hours a week and by 2009, to 48 hours. Pickersgill (2001) claims that this will demand profound changes within healthcare as trainee doctors are concerned over their quality of training and healthcare managers worry about delivering a service which remains largely provided by junior doctors.

Knowledge

Increasing technological and manufacturing change has expanded computer ownership and internet access with broadband connections in the UK quadrupling since 2003. This will have significant implications within the knowledge community and, in relation to accessing specialist health information, will alter the 'information asymmetry' historically found within the patient–practitioner relationship (Newbold, 2005: 444). Muir Gray (1999: 1552) argues that the worldwide web, 'the dominant medium of the post-modern world, has blown away the doors and walls of the locked library' of specialist knowledge. The implications of this for healthcare are significant.

Change in healthcare

The wider social changes noted above can be magnified when applied to healthcare.

Population trends

Despite improvements in population health, across most European countries the growth of an ageing population creates a heavy and profound demand on health and social care services. The eldest group consume proportionately greater health and social services due to increases in chronic and degenerative illnesses. Pressure on costs for informal care within families will rise as the demand for support from these groups increases. The declining trend in birth rates already impacts on the population structure. By 2014 the numbers of older people (over 65) will be above those under 16 (ONS, 2006a), but replacement level fertility, which should be around 2.1 to maintain the population structure is currently at an average of 1.4 across Europe (Smallwood and Chamberlain, 2005).

Other health concerns include a rise in sexually transmitted diseases, drug misuse and teenage pregnancy rates indicating a need for future service development and reconfiguration.

Changing health technologies

These include advances in molecular genetics and their application to human disease as well as advances in techniques of body imaging, microsurgery, transplantation and in the technical ability to sustain life increasing pressure on the costs of long-term care and end-of-life decisions. The introduction and rolling out of such advances create higher expectations from the public. Higher expectations change behaviour and are some of the main drivers of individual and organizational change in the health services. Health professionals too need to change; there are implied requirements of upskilling, improving knowledge to facilitate patient choices between different diagnostic tools, treatment regimes and patient journeys and giving more detailed advice, information and explanations to patients to facilitate choice (Faulkner, 1997).

Prescribing medicines is becoming increasingly challenging. Modern drugs are pharmacologically more complex, the use of poly-pharmacy is growing and increasing iatrogenic morbidity (Aronson et al., 2006). Other emerging concerns centre on the over prescribing of antibiotics and the consequent rise in antibiotic resistant diseases (Magee et al., 1999).

Despite improvements in health, statistics indicate an inexorable rise in prescription rates and costs (see Table 3.1). These concerns have provoked claims of medicine's failure as a modernist project which promised a better world, free of disease and inequality, whereas what has emerged is a profession contributing to ill health (Illich, 1977), unable to provide cures for chronic illnesses and hastening the flight to complementary medicine.

New forms of information transfer

The growth of information technology is having a revolutionary impact on widening access to health knowledge for practitioners and the public. Electronic databases and the National

Table 3.1   Prescribing rates in England

		1997	**2002**	**% increase**
Number of prescription items	(millions)	500	617	23.40
Number of prescription forms	(millions)	287.4	325.5	13.25
Total costs	(millions)	£4919.80	£7161.90	45.57
Average total cost per prescription		£9.80	£11.60	18.36

Source: adapted using data from Hospital and Family Health Services, England and Wales, ONS, 2006b.

electronic Library for Health provide current guidelines and evidence for clinical decisions. The introduction of electronic patient records is planned as part of the health service's modernization project to enable reliable and rapid 24-hour access to records and promote integrated care for all patients by health professionals sharing data. Though their introduction experienced difficulties in acceptance by professionals and concerns over the ethics of access and confidentiality, the system should revolutionize the recording and transmission of test result data and create efficiencies in communication, the patient journey and treatment planning. Internet use has provided increased information for more people; specialist health sites, often disease related, are available for all to download in preparation for health appointments. Social Trends data (ONS, 2006a) indicate the impact of the NHS Direct website: launched in 1999, it contains a comprehensive health encyclopaedia and interactive self-help guide and received an average of 169,000 visits a month in 2001/2 rising to 774,000 by 2004/5 – more than a four-fold increase.

Healthcare delivery

Although the core business of healthcare remains, all types of patient contact and 'episodes of care' have increased, endorsing Dent's (1995) view that the basic premise of the NHS, to free people from illness and disease, turned out to be false, resulting in its continual growth in size and complexity. According to NHS statistics (DH, 2006a) between 1981 and 2004:

- Finished consultant episodes rose from approx 5.7 million to over 8.8 million.
- Length of stay in hospital (excluding day cases) fell from 8.4 days to 4.9 days.
- In-patients per bed more than doubled from 31 to over 68.
- Between 1995 and 2004, hospital admissions increased by almost 2 million (18.6 per cent).

The report indicates that, despite the political rhetoric and management efforts expended to meet waiting time targets, the mean waiting time in 2004/5 (84 days) is only 5 per cent lower than it was in 1995–96.

The Wanless Report (2002) outlines enduring healthcare themes to be addressed: client satisfaction levels; extending choice; improving patient-centred care; reducing waiting times; and dealing with the gap between rising expectations and the everyday reality of patient experience. The report envisions the state of healthcare in 2022 and expects:

1 Large scale relocation of services from hospital to community.
2 Increased patient self care.
3 An integrated information and communication strategy.
4 Greater user involvement in all aspects of care.
5 Integrated referral systems.
6 Faster access – waiting times reduced to 2 weeks for both in- and out-patients.
7 Improved information and access.
8 Progression from 'informed consent' to 'informed choice'.

This new healthcare world view is summarized thus:

> In this vision, patients receive consistently high quality care wherever and whoever they are. It is appropriate, timely and in the right setting. Different types of care are effectively integrated into a smooth, efficient, hassle-free service. With support from the NHS, people increasingly take responsibility for their own health and well-being. Through media such as the internet and digital TV, people receive more information and interactive advice on the management of their and their family's health. (Wanless, 2002: 15)

However, Box 3.1 shows an action research study indicating that such assumptions should be made with caution.

Box 3.1

Overview

Marshall et al. (2006) argue that there is a strong assumption by policy makers that primary care patients behave as consumers and want comparative information to be able to choose between different GP providers. Their study shows that the public are not interested in accessing and using this information.

Aims

To explore the information needs of patients, improve their engagement with practice information and develop an information source about general practice services.

Exploratory and planning phases

Contact with four Primary Care Organizations in UK, 19 GP practices, 103 patients and 49 staff steering groups for data collection via interviews with managers, focus groups with patients and staff, observation, document analysis (annual reports, minutes of meetings), and field notes to examine the drivers and resistors to information development.

(Continued)

(Continued)

Decision and action phase

Results feedback to participants to agree on format for information and key implementers: five main themes generated:

1   Information centred on needs of public not clinicians or policy makers.
2   Hard performance data were not so useful; personal patient feedback was preferable and more trustworthy.
3   Comparative, ranked 'league tables' were disliked – sceptical about reliability.
4   Information was 'politicized'; preferable to have 'many voices' produced through co-operation; decisions regarding 'truth' can be made personally.
5   Information on how the service works and commitments to improvement rather than clinical performance data.

Final phase

Findings used to create a *Guide to General Practice* and a website (www.yourGPguide. org.uk) built on hierarchical needs of patients: context – services – people.

Summary

Patients have different information needs compared to practitioners and do not behave as traditional consumers, often choosing GPs through convenience. They integrate hard performance data and details of service availability and care with their beliefs and experiences. They have strong emotional ties to their doctors.

The basis of change

The above discussion points to several deep and significant changes in the structure and organization of healthcare services in the future.

In setting out his philosophy for modernizing public services, the Prime Minister, in 2002, captured the forces of rising individualism in a freer society and with it, greater demands and expectations of service provision. These provisions are available for many consumer products such as banking and other financial services, supermarkets and leisure pursuits. In an effort to reconcile the culture of individualism and the need for solidarity, he argued that:

> The answer is to move beyond the 1945 settlement because the world has moved beyond the conditions of the immediate post-war era. The 1945 settlement was the social equivalent of mass production when uniformity after decades of the 'welfare lottery' was an entirely worthy ambition. Its aim was to provide a universal, largely basic and standardised service. Individual aspirations were often weak and personal preferences were a low

or non-existent priority … This is no longer true … Today's population generally enjoy choice, quality, opportunity and autonomy on a scale never previously experienced.

We argue the case for moving beyond the outdated mass production approach that too often characterised public services after 1945. (Blair, 2002: 3–4)

The main impetus to moving beyond the 'outdated' systems is the recognition that there is a need to 'give expression to … values in a time of unprecedented aspirations, declining deference and increasing choice, of diverse needs and greater personal autonomy' (Blair, 2002: 9). Hence, in future, public services should be:

characterised by the flexibility, choice and responsiveness that people have grown accustomed to in other parts of their lives … Modern public services need to affirm our status as citizens while meeting our demands as consumers. (Blair, 2002: 19)

In referring to the 1945 settlement as the inflexible social equivalent of 'mass production' and contrasting this with its successor, 'flexibility and choice', Blair recognized that the organization of goods and services had changed during the late twentieth century from what is widely seen as 'Fordism' to its gradual replacement, post-Fordism, to which this discussion will now turn.

Fordism

Precise meanings and qualities concerning Fordism are disputed (Edgell, 2006). It is generally seen as a pattern of social organization embracing features such as the labour process, the economy and social regulation evident through much of the twentieth century. Henry Ford ushered in a manufacturing process that moved away from a traditional system of self-managed, skilled craft workers who assembled a small number of high-quality, non-standard parts into a single product, to a system based on machine tools making standard and interchangeable parts and organized on a rigid but moving assembly line (Edgell, 2006). This transformed the manufacturing process to mass production and mass consumption of standardized consumer durables with demand regulated by supply – a model of 'one size fits all'. The economies of scale reduced production costs and made 'luxury' items widely available, though in a 'standard' way. Work could be done by less skilled and cheaper labour closely controlled by supervisors to ensure time and motion adherence. However, production was fragmented with workers focusing on one small part of the process, using machinery for standardization and simplification, so distancing them from the product. As Edgell summarizes:

Fordism became a short-hand for standardization: a standardized product produced by standardized machinery using standardized methods and standardized human labour employed for a standard working day … also in standardized consumption, and standardized lifestyles, even standardized politics, often referred to as the post-war consensus. (Edgell, 2006: 77/79)

'Fordist' organizations are frequently large, hierarchical and bureaucratic, such as factories, hospitals and the civil service. They tend to be characterized by inflexible work times, tasks and routines. Workers are generally tightly controlled with specifically trained sub-occupations. Their unwieldy communication systems and committee-type structures means services tend to be planned and organized for the benefit of the provider with little input by the user. Actions in response to consumer needs and demands tend to be slow (Walby et al., 1994).

Fordism in healthcare

Walby et al. (1994) claim the obvious example of Fordism in healthcare was the single act of nationalization which created centralized authority and universal, standard provision. They further argue that the system endorses constant sub-division of medical tasks, the development of multiple and specialized health occupations and their relatively narrow training creates workers with a limited range of skills and responsibilities requiring close control by managers. Dent (1995) too, argues that Fordist principles underpin the pyramidal forms of management within hospitals, the wider organization of healthcare, and the emphasis on qualities such as efficiency and effectiveness. Although Mohan (1995) agrees as 'undeniable' that the NHS formed part of the settlement between capital and labour that underpinned Fordism, he cautions that because of the multifaceted nature of Fordism it cannot be assumed that the NHS was ever a Fordist service. He cites, as examples, the difficulty of exercising managerial control over clinicians (see Chapter 4), arguing that key resource decisions have always been made by doctors (Mohan, 2003), and the rise in private healthcare provision and complementary therapies.

Fordist systems, however, endure within healthcare today (Bolton, 2004) through the development of more restrictive contracts for consultants reducing their autonomy, the imposition of targets and 'performance' criteria through medical audit, reduction in treatment decisions through imposing prescribing limitations of generic drugs and the abandoned hospital star-rating system. Collectively, these measures demand Fordist conformity and uniformity.

The critique of Fordism

Dent (1995) claims that during the 1980s it began to be realized that the organizational forms of Fordism were no longer seen as appropriate, particularly the features of hierarchy, centralized planning and control systems and the specialized division of labour. Specifically, the critique of Fordism centred around a slow-down in Western economic growth; the effects of the oil crisis in the early 1970s; an erosion of the West's long term economic superiority over other parts of the world; increasing labour dissatisfaction and industrial action; the unsuitability of Fordist systems in sectors other than manufacturing, particularly where non-standard responses are indicated such as the service sector; the growth in power and demands of the consumer; and the rapid shift in patterns of taste and consumption requiring higher quality, variable and individualized goods – all illustrating the rigidity and limitations of Fordism.

Edgell (2006) argues that Fordism inherently alienates workers and this dissatisfaction adversely affects productivity and profits. Since the 1980s more flexible work systems have been introduced with the downsizing of large industries together with the introduction of new technologies, notably IT systems, allowing the introduction of flexitime, the development of multi-skilled workers and an increase in agency and contracted workers. Edgell (2006) summarizes Fordism's alleged demise as a result of failing to overcome workers' dissatisfaction from the supply side and consumer dissatisfaction from the demand side.

Post-Fordism

If Fordism is characterized by 'rigidity', then post-Fordism (or 'post-bureaucratic' or 'post-industrial' forms of organizations, Jessop, 1994; Edgell, 2006) is marked by 'flexibility'. This flexibility can be seen in the labour process where there are flexible systems (such as production methods, financial systems and forms of consumption), and flexible multi-skilled labour and organization of the workforce.

De-layering and downsizing processes have been employed to make organizations leaner, less hierarchical, more responsive. Production and organization methods are geared towards economies of scope through the desire for a high level of differentiation of goods, services and forms of consumption and hence the need to embrace competition and entrepreneurialism. There is, therefore, an increasing need for new forms of product and service design and a constant need for innovation, customization and privatization (Jessop, 1994).

Post-Fordism has been fuelled by increased personal mobility and the globalization of consumption through the expansion and impact of technology and, specifically, internet use. Dent (1995) also argues that the rapidly changing patterns of consumption closely relate to the growing ascendancy of post-modern tastes. Even though Fordist and post-Fordist modes of organization can and do co-exist despite the tensions between them (Walby et al., 1994), they represent two opposing models of work and sets of values. The values of public service contradict the values of a flexible, market-driven entrepreneurial culture and pose a dilemma for health professionals.

The 'one size fits all' philosophy of Fordism opposes the 'one size fits me' of post-Fordism.

Post-Fordism in healthcare

At the human level, post-Fordism catches the sense that mass assembly lines are not a civilized way to work and it embodies a desire to change and improve tempered by a realization of the limits of a hierarchically driven social system (Walby et al., 1994). Walby et al. set out two contrasting forms of post-Fordism. Firstly the less optimistic variant, seen in the division between core and peripheral services such as cleaning and cooking services which are contracted out to private firms; secondly, the more optimistic variant focusing on customers who define their priorities and expand the need for choice. Edgell (2006) points out that the vertical bureaucracy associated with Fordism is replaced by organization around the task not the process and is characterized by a flat hierarchy, team management and measuring performance by customer satisfaction.

The UK government has expressed its desire to ensure that the public sector does not fall behind the private sector, requiring doctors and dentists to open in evenings and weekends in line with the extended hours of supermarkets (DH, 2000a). A government advisor, Alan Leighton, at the time the chief executive of the supermarket chain Asda, claims 'Traditional working is a thing of the past and a flexible approach is needed' (Frean, 2000).

Foundation Trusts

An example of the move towards post-Fordism in public services is the development of Foundation Trusts which represent a 'profound change in the history of the NHS and the way in which hospital services are managed and provided' (NHS, 2005: 4). They were devised by the Secretary of State for Health (Alan Milburn) following a visit to the Alcorcon hospital in Madrid. In 2002 it was reported that Spain had decentralized its health services – 10 of the 17 regional communities manage their own public health services signalling the effective end of the health ministry in that country. Milburn explains:

> The NHS has great structural weaknesses – not least its top down centralized system that tends to inhibit local innovation and its monolithic structure that denies patients choice. These weaknesses are a product of the health service's history ... For patient choice to thrive it needs a different environment. One in which there is greater plurality in local services which have the freedom to innovate and respond to patients needs. It is an explicit objective of our reforms therefore to encourage greater diversity in provision and more choice for patients ... where different healthcare providers – public, private, voluntary and not-for-profit – work to a common ethos ... healthcare no longer needs to always be delivered exclusively by line managed NHS organisations. (DH, 2002b)

Foundation Trusts, established by The Health and Social Care (Community Health and Standards) Act 2003, appear to embrace post-Fordist and post-modern organizational forms and are seen by their proponents as 'setting the NHS free' (Walshe, 2003: 106). The move from the rigidity of Fordism to the flexibility of post-Fordism can be traced through the arguments for Foundation Trusts which:

- have emerged from a governmental desire to decentralize, devolve decision-making, 'localize' services and hasten a 'patient-led' health service;
- are a new type of 'mutual' organization ensuring community involvement and accountability in the management of local services with the 'freedom' to develop new ways of working reflecting local needs and priorities;

- will be run on 'democratic' principles where local patients, carers and staff can become 'members' and stand for election to the Board of Governors and the Board of Directors responsible for the day-to-day management of services;
- will be free from the direction and control of government and will not be performance managed by Health Authorities (NHS, 2005).

As well as these features, they have a number of restrictions limiting their freedom and serving as a reminder that they are not share-owned, private or competitive companies. So, Foundation Trusts:

- must use their resources to provide NHS services to NHS patients under NHS principles – free and based on clinical need;
- are prevented from building society type demutualization or privatization;
- will operate through an accountability framework to the Board, Commissioners and 'Monitor' (the Independent Regulator of NHS Foundation Trusts);
- cannot make profits and private work is restricted;
- must engage with local communities and co-operate with NHS services.

Post-Fordist principles are underpinned by flexibility and endorse Jessop's prophetic contention that in order to survive, post-Fordist enterprises will have to depend on their capacity to design flexible service delivery and accelerate product and process innovation (Jessop, 1994). 'NHS Foundation Trusts will … use their freedoms to explore innovative approaches to a range of workforce issues, eg. creating new types of jobs, new ways of working and more flexible shift patterns to meet local needs' (NHS, 2005: 13).

The introduction of Foundation Trusts is not without its severe critics on all political sides:

- Fears are centred on the service forming a 'two-tier' system of elite and second rate hospitals and a reduction in the desire to co-operate with other sectors.
- There is nervousness surrounding the dynamics of local membership and the potential in-fighting and vested interests which emerge from 'single issue' groups (Dean, 2003). Trust membership is likely to privilege the articulate and well-off.
- Focus on secondary care diverts attention and funds from primary care, seen as having greater long term significance (Cameron, 2003).
- There are accusations that the scheme is untested, is creeping privatization and echoes the reforms of 'Self-governing Trusts' from the previous Conservative administration (Goodman, 2003).

Alternatively, there are reports that the changes did not go far enough and that hospitals should be allowed to launch, merge and close, in response to local need (Shannon, 2003). Walshe (2003) argues that Foundation Hospitals appear radical and exciting, since, for the first time, they signal a real change between NHS organizations and central government and could promote stability by insulation from political control. He cautions, though, that independence from Westminster does not guarantee good management and governance.

Mohan (2003) expresses concern that Foundation Trusts will denigrate some of the positive aspects of central planning mechanisms and cross-subsidy and allow the government to stress that competition and choice are the only options to improve services. Indeed, he claims that the rejection of the old 'command bureaucracy' is being used to justify policies that go further than those of the previous Conservative government.

Research into the experience of governors at a large, early stage London Foundation Hospital has uncovered further difficulties (King's Fund, 2005). Governors complain that they had little or no influence in how the hospital was run; it was difficult for them to develop a corporate view and they were ill-prepared to contribute to its strategic development. Furthermore, it was reported that they had difficulty in representing and communicating with a large and diverse local urban community. The hospital itself had little idea how new governors should act; one respondent claimed that 'All indications are that we are toothless tigers ... and talking parrots' (King's Fund, 2005: 15).

Primary care

In 2005, the Secretary of State for Health (Patricia Hewitt) issued a challenge to GPs. She said that surgeries have to be more accessible to fit with patients' lifestyles, and that patients should be able to register with more than one GP, at home and at work. She underlined her requirement for flexibility by saying that 'If GPs don't want to lead primary care services then of course we need to go elsewhere'; private healthcare firms noted that clear opportunities were being advanced by the government for them to provide primary care services (Lister, 2005). The point made is that services are provided which meet patients' needs – who or what type of organization provides them is irrelevant.

Similarly Corrigan, a government adviser, argued that the system should be made easier for other providers to enter the market. He aligned GP provision to an independent model:

> There are claims that any extension of primary care services to new independent sector providers would in some way mean a privatisation of primary care. The argument that primary care services should not be run by private companies is odd since, from 1948 to the present, primary care has been developed through a small business, private sector model. Organisationally, GPs are most like partnerships of solicitors ... In this sense primary care is already privatised so it is politically very sloppy to see the entry of another form of private enterprise into the primary care market as privatisation. (Corrigan, 2005: 23)

The new General Medical Services contract came into force in 2004, allowing GPs to opt out of providing 'out-of-hours' cover which was deeply unpopular with them, and some 90 per cent had opted out by 2005. Indeed it has been claimed that the opt-out opportunity was a key negotiation lever in the contract being accepted (National Audit

Office, 2006). The report indicates that in primary care, the out-of-hours provision was a 'maturing market' and is being populated by multiple providers including Primary Care Trusts, co-operatives, mutual organizations, commercial and private organizations and NHS Direct.

The 'Tescoization' of public services – the supermarket solution

In setting out a vision for the reform of public services, the Prime Minister in 2002 underlined the goal of achieving patient choice and the plurality of provision required:

> Choice is an important principle for our reform programme. We need far more choice … People living busy lives want far greater choice of access to the NHS – evening and week-end surgeries, NHS Direct, walk-in centres, and greatly improved A & E departments able to cope with routine incidents quickly … Extending choice in these ways involves new ways of engagement with the voluntary and private sectors. We will intensify this process to expand choice for the many. We are keen to engage more private hospitals and over-seas suppliers. (Blair, 2002: 28–9)

These convictions steadily transfer into concrete features on the map of healthcare and other public service provision:

- Flu vaccinations were first offered by the supermarket Asda in 2002. Singh (2005) reports that Boots, the high street chemist, is working with NHS trusts in areas such as smoking cessation and weight management clinics.
- It is reported that a market could emerge in education and parents would be able to choose between 'chains of schools' in the way shoppers select supermarkets. The plans for schools emerge, according to Reform (2004: para2), from a memo from the Head of the Civil Service (Sir Andrew Turnbull) who argues that 'Our aspiration is to move from a politically driven programme of improving services to a system where customers drive improvements through exercising choice from providers who customise services around their needs'.
- Following a report by the Department of Constitutional Affairs (DCA) which described the legal system as 'outdated, inflexible, over-complex and insufficiently accountable or transparent' (DCA, 2003: para 65) there are government plans to widen the public's access to law firms through a 'one-stop shop' with lawyers and accountants practising together. Termed 'Tesco Law', the proposal would transform the present structure with lawyers' practices setting up in supermarkets to provide services for wills, house purchases and other legal work (*Guardian*, 2003).
- Regarding general practice, the chairman of the General Practitioners Committee of the British Medical Association (BMA) wryly suggests that in 2015:

    > Patients – or customers … are able to receive a whole range of services previously provided in hospitals. Many practices have joined together to run the centres. Others are provided by the private sector, and Tesco Health has extended its franchise with the recent takeover of the failing NHS Direct. (Meldrum, 2006: 46)

Having stated that he believes that crystal ball-gazing carries a high risk of being proved wrong, it was soon reported that the supermarket group J Sainsbury's is preparing to be the first retailer to install GP surgeries in its stores which have pharmacies, claiming that the move into healthcare is a natural fit for its brand (Butler, 2006). A further report confirms the supermarket is opening a flexible and convenient surgery in its Greater Manchester store covering evenings and weekends and seeing up to 70 patients per week. The servicing doctors have set up a separate company 'Doctors in Store' for the venture which is funded by the local Primary Care Trust (PCT) (Hawkes, 2008).

Post-modernism

Much of the foregoing discussion again raises the idea of the 'post-modern' project discussed in Chapter 2 in relation to action research. Here, rather than research, the post-modern 'turn' (Scambler, 2002: 27) is relevant to features of the ongoing transformations within social life, technology, culture and organizations.

Buchanan and Badham (1999: 1) argue that 'the relatively stable, ordered, bounded, predictable, rule-based hierarchical organization today seems an anachronism'. In its place there is emerging the so-called 'post-modern' organization which 'is characterised by fluidity, uncertainty, ambiguity and discontinuity ... boundaries are blurred ... hierarchy is replaced'.

Smart (1993: 14) also links these themes to the 'post-modern condition' characterized by 'a cult of the new, a social and economical context in which innovation and novelty have been promoted, their virtues extolled, often through implied associations with ideas of progress and development'. While recognizing its disputed existence and Buchanan and Badham's features above, Smart (1993) argues that post-modernism includes:

- loss of faith in a single, coherent, linear and progressive account of the world (Muir Gray (1999: 1550) claims that a 'suspicion of science' lies at its core); a breakdown of hierarchies of knowledge;
- lessening of distinctions between elite and mass cultures and, hence, medical and 'lay' people, where the status of the 'expert' is challenged and undermined and the status and views of the 'non-expert' are treated as having an equal validity, importance and 'truth'.

Whether or not this is termed post-modernism, it is undeniable that such changes are escalating and affecting traditional relationships between knowledge, authority and ordinary people. This perhaps reached its zenith in *TIME* magazine's 'Person of the Year, 2006':

> But look ... through a different lens and you'll see another story, one that isn't about conflict or great men. It's a story about community and collaboration on a scale never seen before. It's about the cosmic compendium of knowledge Wikipedia and the million-channel people's network YouTube and the online metropolis MySpace. It's about the many wresting power from the few and helping one another for nothing and how that will not only change the world, but also change the way the world changes ... We're looking at an explosion of productivity and innovation ... For seizing the reins of the global media, for

founding and framing the new digital democracy and beating the pros at their own game, *TIME's* Person of the Year is ... you. (Grossman, 2006: 30–1)

The front cover helpfully provided a mirror.

Post-modernism in healthcare

Dent (1995) identifies a range of features in healthcare which, if they were relevant in 1995 appear to have advanced considerably in the first decade of the twenty-first century. He argues that in the new 'post-modern' world:

- Innovation and flexibility are crucial.
- Inter-disciplinary teams replace functional hierarchy.
- Centrality of market relations 'commodifies' health services.
- The patient–doctor/hospital relationship changes from one of 'supplicant' to 'consumer' and the 'knowledge and authority' of the clinician shifts to the patient (Muir Gray, 1999; Newbold, 2005).
- The imperative of 'consumer' demand replaces rational principles of planning.
- Healthcare provision moves from being a citizen's right to a customer service.
- Medical autonomy reduces.
- 'De-differentiation' in the delivery of healthcare services increases (where the boundaries between science and everyday life erode).

These themes are not only embedded in policy documents such as *Creating a Patient-led NHS* (DH, 2005: 30), where the vision for the NHS is 'user-led services with maximum choice and personalization', and *The Expert Patient* (DH, 2001b), but are promoted as major drivers of the key reforms.

The 'lessening of distinctions' (de-differentiation) and 'the status of the expert' between medical and lay knowledge is raised in relation to living with chronic illness and echoes earlier research into 'meetings between experts' (Tuckett et al., 1985):

> This knowledge and experience held by the patient has for too long been an untapped resource ... The emphasis is beginning to shift ... today's patients with chronic diseases need not be mere recipients of care. They can become key decision-makers in the treatment process. By ensuring that knowledge of their condition is developed to a point where they are empowered to take some responsibility for its management and work in partnership with their health and social care providers, patients can be given greater control over their lives. (DH, 2001b: 5)

As a caveat, the report recognizes and stresses that an Expert Patients Programme is not an 'anti-professional initiative' rather it is based on partnership – the expertise of professionals is seen as no less essential in treating chronic disease when patients are involved in self-management.

The aim in *Creating a Patient-led NHS* (DH, 2005: 16) is to build a service which 'continuously adapts to what patients choose'. The 'breakdown in hierarchies of knowledge' and 'rise in consumer demand' raised earlier are evidenced in the power and control being shifted from health professionals to patients who 'will have an informed choice of treatment options, treatment providers, location for receiving care, type of ongoing care and choice at the end of life' (2005: 20). The questions remain however as to whether information is sufficient for patients to make decisions, whether they want to (see Box 3.1), whether they are able to, and the consequences when there are the inevitable disagreements between customer and provider.

Flexible staff

In this new world of innovation and flexibility, staff are not forgotten as they will be given 'more autonomy and authority to act' (DH, 2005: 24). It is claimed that the problems derived from the worst aspects of the health service (hierarchical tradition; professional divides; bureaucratic systems; inflexible processes) will reduce with:

> the increase in multi-disciplinary working, new staff contracts which promote flexibility, new roles for many staff groups, new technologies, choice and contestability and, in places, much more entrepreneurial behaviours. Patients will demand more flexible services. Staff will quickly need to offer more flexible responses. (DH, 2005: 24)

Walshe provides a counterbalancing view when he claims that:

> none of this bewildering succession of health service reforms has changed the fundamental governance and accountability arrangements of the NHS. The service remains, just as it was when it was founded in 1948, a vertically integrated public bureaucracy run from Whitehall. (Walshe, 2003: 108)

Box 3.2 shows a study where the benefits of collaborative working and reducing boundaries benefits patients' safety.

Box 3.2

Overview

Mitchell et al. (2005) report on a study from Northern Ireland to improve the knowledge and skills of nurses in moving and handling stroke patients and introduce safer practices in a rehabilitation unit.

The 'trigger' was a member of staff who encountered a nurse and physiotherapist attempting to manually transfer a patient with hemiplegia in contravention of agreed protocols (hoist use). The action was halted to prevent potential damage and thus emerged an urgent need to ensure that patient handling was consistent with regulations. The aims of the project were:

(i) to facilitate nurses in sharing insights into moving and handling patients;
(ii) to enable nurses to identify facilitators of this practice;
(iii) to empower nurses and physiotherapists to direct changes in their practice.

Exploratory and planning phase

A literature review was undertaken which showed that:

- Nurses continue to manually lift patients incorrectly.
- Nurses display negative attitudes to changing practice.
- Nurses conform to unsafe practice to avoid negative reactions.
- Equipment was often faulty and contaminated.
- Team-working positively influenced safer patient handling practice.
- Nurses felt that physiotherapists had little respect for their knowledge base.
- Physiotherapists found that nurses were reluctant to follow their advice.

Three focus group meetings were held where staff aired their views and insights into manual handling practice which were recorded and fed back by researchers. Findings indicated:

- There were concerns that using hoists could hinder rehabilitation.
- Manual handling guidance can conflict with promoting independence.
- Junior staff felt pressure to conform.
- Nurses felt they had insufficient detail on patients' progress when attending physiotherapy.

Brainstorming sessions focused on actions that would assist staff to use the hoist. Findings were summarized and fed back to staff and included:

- Additional hoists with weighing devices and extra slings.
- More space around the beds and more time to use hoists correctly.
- Problems with electrical cables under beds.
- Greater collaborative working with physiotherapists.

Decision and action phase

A consensus was reached over the following actions:

- Purchase of new 'weighing' hoist, an additional 'lifting' hoist, and extra slings and sliding sheets.
- Training for equipment use through company demonstration.
- Senior staff to address problems of peer pressure.
- Greater collaboration between physiotherapists and nurses – physiotherapists and nurses conducted daily updates on patients' handling needs.
- Electrical cables were referred to the Trust's clinical effectiveness coordinator.

Second observation/reflection phase

- Nurses reported problems with a hoist which was corrected.
- Senior nurses were supervising junior staff.
- Nurses and physiotherapists were updating each other regularly.

(Continued)

(Continued)

A later phase of reflection by nursing staff identified three themes:

- Empowerment – staff felt involved, valued and confident.
- Changing practice – staff had learned correct processes through their involvement.
- Collaboration – all staff became involved and, through this, understanding between physiotherapists and nurses was enhanced.

Summary

Clinical practice can be changed in a multi-disciplinary setting where openness and collaboration are used and participants are involved in directing and evaluating proposed changes.

Conclusion

To achieve the current aspirations staff at all levels will need much more devolved power and authority to take decisions and should have the incentives to implement change within their sphere of responsibility. The current health policy context implies a need for new financial regimes with far less central planning and greater opportunity for local decisions based on local needs. In theory, practitioners will require more local knowledge of financial flows of commissioners' and providers' resources to ensure that any proposed service is properly budgeted and managed within cost constraints. In practice, however, no single practitioner can take decisions based solely on individual patient choice or demands, especially where services have a public health bias.

Chapter summary

- The world is changing rapidly. The main influences include globalization, lifestyle trends, health concerns, organization of labour and increased knowledge management.
- Healthcare provision needs to respond to changes in population trends, health technologies, information transfer and new forms of health delivery.
- These influences have prompted moves from Fordist to post-Fordist and post-modern forms of organizations though these face difficulties when applied to healthcare.
- In healthcare, these trends promote greater freedom, independence, flexibility, a breakdown in traditional boundaries and an increase in patient choice.
- Flexible delivery and roles threaten traditional ways of working and the provision of a national service.

4

Management in Healthcare: Theory and Practice

Introduction

Chapter 2 discussed the influence and importance of the Industrial Revolution in the transition to the 'modern' era which heralded a significant period of social, economic and technological change, particularly in the organization of labour. In pre-modern times, most work was non-industrial and unregulated, occurring mainly in rural communities involved with farming and other agricultural related pursuits. Work was located within families and households, which were both the means of production and consumption with little gender differentiation (Edgell, 2006). Goods were produced manually by skilled or semi-skilled craft workers working individually, co-operatively or in cottage industries, where payment was in cash or kind and commuting any distance was unknown. In these situations there was limited need for controls or a management class. 'Pre-modern' artisans exercised self-management with some autonomy over their work conditions determining the volume, pace and payment rates of work undertaken.

Social change does not occur in a vacuum, and technological developments throughout the Industrial Revolution enabled the widespread mechanization of the manufacturing process notably in the textile, pottery, glass, mining and metal industries. Migration of workers to cities fuelled the rapid development and expansion of factory based production. Concentrations of large numbers of workers meant there needed to be changes to systems of management and control in order to maintain or raise productivity and reduce costs, particularly as factory owners viewed workers as little more than commodities (Marsh, 2000). Furthermore, in contrast to the 'whole product' approach of earlier artisans, industrial workers increasingly worked on a specific part or task within a more extensive manufacturing process. A new type of employee, the 'manager' or supervisor (literally an 'over-seer') emerged as an agent of capital accumulation responsible for regulating workers' performance. Managerial activities began to be conceived separately from those of workers to achieve improvements in the direction, organization and co-ordination of labour activities and the control and support of those who had to be managed. Thus began the proliferation of management schools and theories, each claiming a distinct, different and 'new' approach.

The discipline of management has been criticized for its eagerness to reject older theories (and theorists) in favour of the latest 'innovative' idea potentially causing it to 'implode under the weight of its own contradictions' (Hales, 2001: 52). This has led to seminal theorists being stereotyped as old fashioned and outdated in order to privilege the latest fad. As Grint has summarized 'management fads and fashions seem to change with the seasons and what counts as common sense one year will undoubtedly prove to be self-evident claptrap the following year' (1995: 2).

This chapter discusses some historical changes in management within healthcare before considering two areas of theory; 'classical/scientific', and 'human relations'. It will conclude by identifying and integrating key managerial concepts into a practical 'approach to management' for health professionals (Figure 4.1).

The major concepts of the model shown in Figure 4.1 have been developed using the method outlined by Zuber-Skerritt (2002: 143):

- identifying core categories and issues from the literature;
- identifying sub-categories;
- mapping/patterning relationships between categories into a two- or three-dimensional diagram;
- experimenting, obtaining feedback and revising/refining the representation.

Managing healthcare

'Old' management

Goodwin (2006) maintains that the current contextual challenges facing healthcare (see Chapter 3) are so complex that they defy simple solutions. The essential task for healthcare management in the early 1970s was to 'organise limited resources – human, financial and physical – to enable the community to be provided with the best possible standard and balance of care. This entails establishing priorities between conflicting claims' (DHSS, 1972b: 14).

The goal of health management is similar today:

> Effective management … underlies the delivery of safe, effective and patient-focused healthcare services. The importance of management is underlined by the fact that the most consistent message to emerge from our investigations of serious service failures in the NHS is that failures in leadership and management can have devastating consequences for patients. Managers of services cannot plan for the long term future of services in isolation. They need to involve staff … as well as patients and the public. Some still need to involve clinicians and other staff more to ensure they can deliver further improvements. (Healthcare Commission, 2006: 93)

The need for effective management in large, pluralistic and bureaucratic healthcare organizations is immense because of the different vested interests, the variety of political, professional, administrative and lay goals and the resulting set of competing and often incompatible rationalities which have to be managed effectively. Strategies used in the past to accommodate the professional 'vested interests' attempted, through the administration of multiple interlocking committees (the cogwheel system) and consensus management, to involve all practitioners, particularly doctors, to manage their work systematically and develop their managerial abilities (Hunter, 1991). The professionally driven service of the 1950s to1980s gave rise to various coalitions termed 'practitioner interest' and 'administrative interest' (Thompson, 1987). These coalitions however produced areas of conflict when attempting to achieve service goals (Freidson, 1990). One continuing area of conflict is medicine's claims for clinical autonomy. This developed from the primacy of medical knowledge, the prestige of its professional status, control over technology and the uniqueness of the doctor–patient relationship. Tolliday argues that doctors have clinical autonomy because, although state provided, the delivery of healthcare is 'personalised' which 'gives doctors a right to unmanaged status' (1976: 37). The allopathic healthcare mentality and the belief that disease has a unique individual biological base have led successive governments to support individualized rather than population-based healthcare systems (Hunter, 1992). Clinicians' Hippocratic ideology is necessarily individualized (and sometimes idiosyncratic, Davies and Harrison, 2003) in trying to achieve the best care for their patients. This is termed 'possessive individualism' (Hunter, 1994: 12) and perpetuates notions of elitism even within collegiate relationships.

In contrast to the 'practitioner interest', the 'administrative ethic' is built on the concept of formal rationalism or bureaucratization, a rational-legal system of authority whose power base is derived from the application of information systems and administrative procedures and protocols. Bureaucratization developed from the drive for centralization and Fordist economies of scale thereby allowing claims of quality and efficiency. Officials of the bureaucratic market control which goods and services are produced (Freidson, 1990). In healthcare, control of resources was ensured by 'countering the accepted status of clinical autonomy with the pervasiveness of objective information and rational argument' (Thompson, 1987: 139). The administrative ethic enabled health services to function through facilitation and support rather than taking an active management role. This led to criticisms that:

- The balance of supply and demand lay in the hands of health professionals.
- There were reduced incentives for economies.
- There was potential for waste and inefficiency.
- There were higher costs and longer waits for treatments as practitioners pursued their own ends.

'New' management

Dent (1993) reports that by the 1980s the demands and costs of healthcare provision had risen to such a level that more effective methods had to be devised to control and contain them. Following the 'Griffiths' inquiry into the management of the NHS (DHSS, 1983) the notion of 'new rationalism' was introduced which reflected the phenomenon of 'managerialism' (Hunter,1992) which was pervading society.

The inquiry argued that the health service needed a cultural change rather than merely another reorganization and, by introducing general management and business practices it attempted to re-define the decision-making process at all levels.

Through the appointment of 'general managers', Griffiths dismissed the notion of a 'gentleman's agreement' for decision making through negotiation (Scrivens, 1988: 1754) which had led to 'lowest common denominator decisions ... the absolute need to get agreement overshadowed the substance of the decision required' (DHSS, 1983: 17, 22). Griffiths explicitly criticized the administrative ethic yet clearly defined the rational management process which remains prevalent today:

> One of our most immediate observations from a business background is the lack of a clearly defined management function throughout the NHS. By general management, we mean the responsibility drawn together in one person ... for planning, implementation and control of performance ... Absence of this general management support means that there is no driving force seeking and accepting direct and personal responsibility for developing management plans, securing their implementation, and monitoring actual achievement ... above all ... a lack of a *general management process* means that it is extremely difficult to achieve change. (DHSS, 1983: 11, my emphasis)

Managers were no longer to be supporters of health professionals but were empowered for both operational and strategic decision making. They became a new, separate and non-clinical group whose role was to control health professionals (Thorne, 1997). Healthcare management therefore developed into a distinctly different activity from the clinical work of health professionals.

Managerialism

Managerialism was criticized as lacking sensitivity to the caring aspects of health work (Currie, 1998) and exposed the incompatibility of managerially determined targets with the essence of professional practice (Winyard, 2003).

Managerialism comprises a set of beliefs and practices, at the core of which is the assumption that better management will prove an effective solution for a wide range of personal, economic and social ills (Pollitt, 1993) and has been promoted in healthcare by successive governments. The techniques of managerialism demand the setting of targets and priorities, analysing activities, monitoring and appraising performance against set criteria, setting and controlling budgets and workforce targets and implementing management information systems (Pollitt, 1993). It has been linked to attempts to privatize, commercialize and de-regulate public sector services (Pollock, 2005) and has been criticized as being inappropriate for the organizational complexities and ethos of public services (Thorne, 1997). These requirements call for clear leadership and management skills

Table 4.1   Perceived differences between practitioners and managers

Doctors/Practitioners	Managers
• Rooted in biological science	• Draws from economics, finance, social and behavioural sciences
• Direct cause/effect relationships	• Less clear cause/effect relationships
• Strong academic rigour	• Weak rigour in strategy/marketing
• Strong evidence base (e.g. Cochrane)	• Weak evidence-based management
• Strong written culture	• Weak written culture
• Ancient colleges and specialist groups	• Short professional life-span
• Senior doctors work with patients	• Senior managers remote from customers
• Responsible for own individual patients	• Focus on groups and populations
• Professional discretion in treatment decisions	• Decisions based on rational/legal policy
• Think operationally	• Think strategically
• Work to short time frames	• Plan for longer time horizons
• Individualistic characteristics and uneasy with being led	• Work generally in teams
• Tendency to dominate teams	• More comfortable with conflict and negotiation
• Operate within a professional culture	• Operate in a task or role culture

Sources: Thorne (1997); Ferlie and Shortell (2001); Smith (2003b).

Table 4.2   Principal concerns of practitioners and managers

Doctors/Practitioners	Managers
• Patient/client outcomes	• Patient experience
• Focus on individual patients/clients	• Emphasis on populations/organization
• Optimum care for each patient/client	• Trade-offs between competing claims
• Need for professional autonomy	• Need for public accountability
• Desire for self-regulation	• Preoccupied with systems
• Use of evidence-based practice	• Fair allocation of resources
• Tendency to personal responsibility	• Tendency to delegation

Source: adapted from Edwards et al. (2002, 2003).

but also stricter controls over professional decision making and activities and hence a curtailing of clinical freedom and professional autonomy. This is the 'hub and the rub' of health service management (Scrivens, 1988: 1754) where the 'fundamental problem is a paradox between calls for a common set of values and the need to recognize that doctors and managers do and think differently' (Edwards et al., 2003: 609). There are deep differences in doctors' and managers' backgrounds (Table 4.1) illustrated by the study in Box 4.1, and their different concerns (Table 4.2) give rise to 'unavoidable conflict between the reductionist approach of medicine and the messy, political and complex world of policy' (Edwards et al., 2002: 837).

Box 4.1

Overview

Shani and Eberhardt (1987) report on a study to understand and improve healthcare team effectiveness in a Medical Rehabilitation Hospital (MRH). Differences were found between two major teams, one managed by a physician (clinical) and another by a case manager (administrative). Discrepancies were found in areas of functioning (structures, processes and effectiveness) and the spoken philosophy underlining their orientation.

Problem identification

- Team members and senior management did not have a shared understanding of teamwork.
- The reality of teamwork differed from the philosophy imposed by senior management.
- Previous attempts by senior management to improve teamwork design and effectiveness failed.
- An approach without management control was required.
- Action research using practitioners' understanding of teamwork was deemed most appropriate.

Planning and data collection methods

A 'parallel' organization was planned to become a 'microcosm of the medical organizational subsystem' (Shani and Eberhardt, 1987: 154) as the experimental vehicle to examine teamwork effectiveness. Organizational ideas were collected, shared and acted on which enhanced organizational learning.

Staff members were selected to make up the 'parallel' organization.

Meetings were held with senior management to create the foundations of a 'learning' climate and set the scope of the study:

- interviews with selected staff;
- survey questionnaire on staff attitudes ($n=158$, 78 per cent) regarding the organizational context;
- compilation of themes from interviews;
- summary of results and feedback.

Results and decision phase

- Thirty 'issues' were associated with team characteristics with 14 dominant themes.
- Participants showed hostility towards management's unresponsiveness to suggestions for improvements.
- The parallel organization created a climate of trust, openness and co-inquiry but this was not reflected throughout the hospital.
- Data showed problems related to physicians' behaviour and managers' styles.

- More effective teams shared expectations and minimal discrepancies between actual and expected work team conditions. The hospital's size, history and conditions affected teamwork.
- Clinical teams felt they were 'multi-disciplinary' rather than 'interdisciplinary'. Team effectiveness was influenced by team dynamics which was influenced by expectations and discrepancies determined by the hospital context.

Implementation phase

The parallel organization proposed three solutions:

1 Massive change programme for hospital-wide redesign to create unified teams.
2 Piecemeal change based on recommendations and managements priorities (though not as radical as 1).
3 Scientific longitudinal study to compare effectiveness of multi- and inter-disciplinary teams.

Decisions

The medical director recognized that plan 1 was superior but felt that only a scientific study would convince physicians of the need to change and this was consequently created.

Summary

The parallel organization is an action research method to tap into and integrate members' organizational knowledge to arrive at new understandings. Members learnt more skills, engaged in a greater variety of activities, carried out more tasks and experienced more autonomy and independence. As the parallel organization matured, the formal organization's mission, strategy, design and processes were questioned more deeply.

Davies et al. (2003) report that, of the main groups of senior doctors in management, clinical directors are the most disaffected, with many holding negative views of managers' abilities, the balance of power between them and any prospects for improved working relations.

Perhaps the key to understanding role conflicts is what Fitzsimmons and White (1997: 126) term the 'internal orientation' in medicine, described as 'the doctor, patient and the illness'. They argue that general practitioners' one-to-one orientation conflicts with a wider service perspective towards the general population, their health needs and effective use of finite resources which are the legitimate concern of managers who must hold a collective view (Degeling and Carr, 2004).

There are also important similarities (Table 4.3) where managers and clinical practitioners can and should learn from each other (Smith, 2003b) but patients, Edwards et al. (2003) claim, are best served by the continued tension between the two.

Table 4.3   Similarities between managers and practitioners

- Extended and continual training
- Concern for ethics
- Respond to financial incentives
- Action oriented
- Opportunities to specialize
- Reputations as poor communicators
- Engage in excessive use of jargon
- Engage in breaking bad news
- Encourage people to change
- Lack of women and ethnic minorities in senior positions

Source: Smith (2003b).

Effects on health professionals

Doctors

The move to managerialism together with more general changes in perceptions of power and authority in society, mount a significant challenge to the traditional position of the expert, particularly in medicine, and raise questions concerning the extent of its deprofessionalization and proletarianization. There is a considerable volume of historical literature which analyses medicine as a profession and its ability to exercise occupational dominance (Freidson, 1970; Haug, 1988; Elston, 1991; Kelleher et al,. 1994; Harrison and Ahmed, 2000), seen as the 'authority to direct and control the work of others without in turn being subject to direction and evaluation by them' (Freidson, 1970: 135). Elston (1991: 61) categorizes three types of professional autonomy:

- Economic autonomy – the right to determine remuneration.
- Political autonomy – the right to make policy decisions.
- Technical autonomy – the right to set clinical standards and performance.

Kelleher et al. (1994) and Edwards et al. (2002) agree that in the developed world, medicine has become both deprofessionalized and proletarianized. Deprofessionalization has occurred through the 'secularization of medical mystique' (Kelleher et al., 1994: xiii), the narrowing of the knowledge gap via the use of the internet (see Chapter 3), the rise and incorporation into mainstream healthcare of alternative therapies, and the encroachment of Allied Health Professions on practice areas. An example of this can be found in the discussion document for the report, *Direction of Travel of Urgent Care* (DH, 2006b) where non-medical teams such as Emergency Care Practitioners are encouraged to provide frontline care and assessment of patients. In its response, the BMA states that:

> Such services are increasingly based on non-medically qualified staff while GPs are disregarded … to remove urgent care from general practice will lead to GPs losing their traditional 'gatekeeper' role and becoming de-skilled … The government needs to listen to the professionals rather than policy apparatchiks if they want to develop coherent change. (BMA, 2007)

Proletarianization occurs through the 'divesting of control over certain prerogatives relating to the location, content and essentiality of its task activities and is therefore subordinated to the broader requirements of production under advanced capitalism' (McKinlay and Arches, 1985 cited in Elston, 1991: 63). This process of limiting professional discretion, and the resistant attitudes towards it, is illustrated by an impassioned letter to *The Times*:

> As a single-handed specialist clinician in the NHS I have six managers: line manager, clinical manager, finance manager, audit manager, department manager, human resources manager.
>
> I will willingly donate a few then I could get on with treating patients ... which is what the NHS is about. (Reay, 2004)

Smith argues 'Doctors are losing out in modern healthcare systems because of their discomfort with leadership, strategy, systems thinking, negotiation, genuine team working, organizational development, economics and finance' (Smith, 2003b: 611). Smith suggests that learning about these management concepts may make doctors 'less lost' in modern healthcare but that managers should learn from doctors about creating an evidence base, engaging in debates about research and getting closer to patients. The persistence of these tensions and deepening bureaucratization compound a lack of awareness of the contribution of other professions, particularly nurse managers (Degeling et al., 2003).

Nurses

Nurses have always had a management function within health services but this has tended to be at the operational level within 'consensus' management rather than the strategic level (Bolton, 2004). Furthermore, managerial efforts were mainly focused on nurse education, the organization and deployment of the nursing workforce and the line management roles of 'training, organizing and monitoring junior nurses' work' (Bolton, 2003: 123) rather than crossing any professional boundaries (Walby et al., 1994). The Griffiths Report was designed to change and manage doctors but the nursing contribution was ignored, even removing their right to a place on management boards (DHSS, 1983). This 'shut out' nursing from managing in the reorganized service (Davies, 1995: 163), though Davies highlights other contributory factors such as the gendered nature of nursing work, nurses' lack of knowledge of leadership, questions over competence, the defensiveness and uncertainty of nurse managers and 'a failure to acknowledge that there was a management job to be done' (1995: 165).

The *NHS Plan* provides some rehabilitation for nurse managers through recreating the modern matron, though the term 'matron' is traditionally gendered and appears out of place in a 'modernization' agenda (Hewison, 2001). The *Plan* sets out '10 key roles' for nurses 'to take a lead in the way local health services are organized and in the way that they are run' (DH, 2000a: 83–4).

It claims that the public consultation provoked a strong call for:

> A 'modern matron' figure – a strong clinical leader with clear authority at ward level ...
> They will be in control of the necessary resources to sort out the fundamentals of care,

backed up by appropriate administrative support ... without getting bogged down in bureaucracy. (DH, 2000a: 86, 135)

Their role is to lead by example, ensure quality of care, clean wards and good food, respect for patients and to resolve problems – though these remain operational rather than strategic (Hewison, 2001).

Outside hospitals, community matrons were discussed in the *NHS Improvement Plan* (DH, 2004a) though their particular focus is on delivering more technological treatment to patients with complex clinical needs. Bolton (2003) points out that government literature avoids using the term 'management', preferring 'leadership' and 'coordination'. Her study provides evidence that nurses wish to disassociate themselves from the term 'manager' and its implications. One respondent states 'I don't want to be seen as a manager. I want to be seen as a leader. These nurses are professionals ... they don't need managing. I want to be more of a facilitator and coordinator' (Bolton, 2003: 126). Another states that the management role 'was a hard faced one' indicating the cultural differences between the professional clinical role in nursing as 'strongly feminised' and management as 'equally strongly masculinised' (Reedy and Learmonth, 2000: 154). This leads to devaluing of clinical nursing knowledge in opposition to 'management knowledge' (Reedy and Learmonth, 2000: 161).

Sambrook (2006: 58) also discusses the transitional difficulties of nurses moving into management, the assault on the nursing identity as 'caring' and the (contested) assumption that 'if you're a nurse you're not very good at business'. Participants in Currie's (1998) study disagree that managerial and clinical skills are interchangeable. At the heart of this dilemma is the belief that there is an incompatibility between the characteristics of management and the essential identity of professional clinical practice creating a clash of ideologies (Reedy and Learmonth, 2000). Managers in Sambrook's study attempt to solve this by changing ward sisters' titles to 'ward manager' in recognition of the 'extra management duties'.

Autonomy plays an important role in nurses' job satisfaction and retention, though Mrayyan (2004: 333) reports that, similarly to doctors, nurses retain more autonomy over patient care decisions as 'managers of patient care' than over unit operations such as selecting staff and budget planning. Mrayyan argues that 'supportive and participative management' significantly increases autonomy in contrast to 'autocratic/non-participative management' which most strongly hinders it, highlighting the vital role that management style has in promoting professional practice.

Analysing terminology

Management

There is no agreement on definitions of management; indeed, there are so many dimensions and theoretical perspectives that to attempt a definition would be fruitless. Discussions need to represent the multidimensional perspectives and ambiguities of managerial work since it can include a spectrum of roles from company directors and chief executives to supervisors at a shop-floor level.

It is difficult to avoid being teleological (an explanation of a phenomenon by reference to its purpose) when discussing the various theoretical and practical terms, but Grint (1995) writes that it derives from the Italian '*maneggiare*' meaning to 'control', from the Latin, '*manus*', the hand, and hence to the 'mundane' meaning of management, 'to handle' a situation or thing (Grey, 2005: 53). Although there is no consensus and terminology is contested, modern definitions see 'management' as the method, or process through which the members of an organization attempt to co-ordinate their activities and use their knowledge, skills and resources to fulfill the various tasks and goals of the organization as efficiently and effectively as possible (Morgan, 1998). This entails balancing and co-ordinating the interests and needs of all employees so that they can work together within the constraints set by the organization's capacity, culture and environment. Drucker synchronizes the main concepts: 'The fundamental task of management remains the same: to make people capable of joint performance through common goals, common values, the right structure, and the training and development they need to perform and to respond to change' (1989: 214). Drucker aligns management with change which Paton and McCalman (2000) see as being synonymous.

Operational management is concerned with shorter term decision making, and routine, day-to-day problem solving, responses to activities, and issues such as staffing levels, scheduling work, ensuring quality, customer relations and staff training. This level may be covered by middle managers, team leaders and supervisors – the nurse managers discussed in the *NHS Plan* (DH, 2000a).

Strategic management is valued more than operational management and concerns larger scale and longer term plans and objectives, making major decisions in the nature, direction, emphasis and structure of the organization (Stoney, 2001). It involves taking a more corporate approach and is concerned with resource allocation, mission development and performance review and reward and is generally undertaken at senior and executive levels. Particularly it concerns positioning the organization within the changing external political and policy environment (Fitzsimmons and White, 1997) (see Figure 4.1).

In public sector organizations, management is focused on ensuring that limited resources are used effectively and services are provided equitably and at the right cost and delivered to an agreed standard, which is acceptable to clients, practitioners and governing bodies.

These statements however make no allowance for variables such as the:

- size and type of organization;
- product being manufactured or service provided;
- market environment in which it operates;
- size and level of competition;
- extent of differentiation and specialisation in employees' skills and knowledge;
- style, power and values of its leaders;
- strength and character of its culture;
- methods of communication;

- extent of rules and regulations governing employee activities;
- prevailing national legislation.

These variables are highly significant and affect the overall achievement of goals. At the ideological level, Harding (1998) argues that 'management' is a belief system which claims that it is an absolute necessity and a vital function peopled by rational-technical functionaries who posses a body of knowledge and skills without which organizations could not survive.

Managers

Handy (1993) has cautioned that it has never been easy to define who managers are or what they do – definitions of the manager, and the manager's role, tend to be so broad that they are meaningless.

Mindful of this caveat, the consistent evidence (Hunt, 1992; Hales, 1999: 342; Hales, 2001: 51) indicates common and broad characteristics of most managers as being:

- a specific group of employees who are separate from 'workers';
- responsible for dealing with the organization and administration of management activities and wider systems of planning, monitoring and control;
- required to promote and maintain order, discipline and structure in areas where activities are undertaken;
- engaged in various levels of strategic and operational decision making which affect the actions and output of workers and the course and direction of organizations;
- accountable for actions in the area of work where they are responsible.

Hales generalizes managers' daily preoccupations as concerned with monitoring and maintaining people, information and work processes and describes the characteristics of these activities as being:

- short, interrupted and fragmented;
- reactive to events, problems and needs of others;
- preoccupied with urgent, ad hoc and unplanned issues;
- multidimensional rather than separate and bounded;
- face-to-face and verbally interactive;
- tense, pressured and conflict ridden in dealing with competing demands;
- open to negotiation over the ways and means of achievement.

These findings have led Harvey-Jones (1990) to claim that middle managers are caught between the upper and lower grindstones where, because of the impact of day-to-day 'troubleshooting' they are unable to concentrate on more strategic and longer term plans and projects. In contrast, Currie (2000: 18) argues that 'implementing strategy' is seen as the 'key strategic role' of middle managers.

In healthcare, however, Michie and West (2004) report there is little medical or nursing research that focuses on work context, people management or employee relations.

Managing

'Managing' is a ubiquitous activity and umbrella term denoting many commonplace, commonsense and everyday activities and skills that most people undertake most of the time – especially those with parental responsibilities (Grint, 1995). It is a process view of the way activities are organized (Thorne, 1997). In other words, in order to 'manage' an activity, project or group, an individual is not required to be designated either as a 'manager' or be part of an organization's formal system of 'management' but yet will carry out many 'management' type actions. These activities are similar throughout all organizational levels and apply to the majority of health professionals at patient/client care, project, unit and corporate/strategic level (Figure 4.1).

Theoretical approaches to management

Although there are innumerable management theories in the literature, two will be discussed here.

Firstly, 'classical/scientific' management as it,

- underpins much contemporary management practice (Lemak, 2004);
- is the traditional approach in healthcare settings (Walby et al., 1994; Bolton, 2004).

Secondly, the 'human relations' approach as it,

- is the aspirational approach of 'new nursing' (Wigens, 1997);
- supports action research and contemporary change management.

Classical/scientific theories

Although the main thrust of industrialization began in England (Marsh, 2000), it spread rapidly to the United States where the mechanization process was applied extensively and successfully in automobile manufacturing. Famously, Henry Ford constructed the mass production assembly line for the Ford model T, introduced in 1908, and fulfilled his ambition of producing a cheap and reliable car for the masses. To meet demand, the 'continuous moving assembly line' was introduced in 1914 and by 1918 half of all cars in America were Ford model Ts (Hounshell, 1984). Commenting on the application of the assembly line to car production, Womack et al. claim that it 'Changed our most fundamental ideas about how we make things. And how we make things dictate not only how we work but what we buy, how we think, and the way we live' (1990: 11).

At the same time as Henry Ford changed his production methods, another American engineer, Frederick Taylor, was concerned with improving worker efficiency in the steel industry. Taylor published one of the first books on management, *The Principles of*

Scientific Management, in 1911 and it was used by Ford in 1914 (Edgell, 2006). At the same time an experienced French engineer, Henri Fayol published his *General and Industrial Management* in 1916, part of which dealt with the 'elements' or 'functions' of management. Since these two theorists were both engineers, there is little surprise that their systems are seen as 'mechanistic'.

They propose management systems which focus on the individual and believe that:

- The rational worker's motivation is driven by economic and promotional incentives.
- Managers' primary aims are to improve efficiency and observe and supervise staff.
- Managers' main roles are to plan the work and control and train staff.

Frederick Taylor (1856–1915)

Taylor (1911/1967) claims that management is a process which emphasizes the separation of the design of work (rational planning and organizing) from its execution, thereby establishing the need for a chain of command, co-ordination of procedures and control of systems.

Control of workers in Taylor's model is through appropriate task allocation aligned to the worker's skills, time and motion study of tasks, and reward for successful performance. Taylor (1911/1967) argues that the role of management is to develop a scientific approach to work – replacing 'rule of thumb' methods with a precise 'scientific' determination of tasks to find the 'one best way'.

Taylor argues that the most prominent element in modern management is the 'task idea' – the work of every employee is fully planned and controlled, with instructions on the task to be accomplished, the means to be used and the time taken (1911/1967: 39). These approaches are found within the design and management of healthcare organizations today (Brooks, 2006) and cause Walby et al., (1994: 137) to claim that 'nurses are currently closest in organization to the Taylorist model'. Bolton also finds Taylorism in nursing work:

> Nurses ... continually point to increasing bureaucratization as evidence that management is now a much more deliberate activity which has resulted in an increase in apparently Taylorist modes of work measurement. Practice protocols, for instance, which give step by step detail of how nursing tasks should be carried out. (Bolton, 2004: 323)

At its simplest, Taylor sees managers' roles as enabling workers to work better and quicker than before.

Henri Fayol (1841–1925)

Henri Fayol, wrote his 'universal principles of management', which Lemak (2004) calls the first comprehensive theory of management, when he was aged 75. He sees management as a continuous process involving five key interdependent functions

(Fayol, 1984; Wren et al., 2002). These share similarities with Taylor's principles and emphasize:

1   Prevoyance (planning and forecasting) – using foresight and setting goals; providing for the future to ensure their achievement.
2   Organizing – ensuring the organization has all the resources it requires to operate successfully, including human, material, finance, space, equipment and time.
3   Command – directing and controlling staff.
4   Co-ordination – conducting and harmonizing activities for successful results.
5   Control – ensuring that methods and systems adhere to the plan.

These approaches stress discipline, authority and responsibility as well as *esprit de corps* (Smith and Boyns, 2005), yet Fayol's key function was 'planning' which entails looking to the future and deciding which actions should be taken to minimize uncertainty.

Although scientific and classical approaches are unfashionable, stereotyped and criticized for being authoritarian, centralizing and promoting uniformity (Eastman and Bailey, 1994; Parker and Ritson, 2005) there is evidence that they are increasing in modern organizations (Pruijt, 2000; Bolton, 2004). Lemak (2004) argues that they are much maligned and it is incorrect to assume that all 'classical' theories are based on task-oriented, anti-worker ideas. Indeed, in offering incentives to workers which include 'better surroundings and working conditions', Taylor (1911/1967: 34) explicitly states that the manager should ensure that incentives should be 'accompanied by … personal consideration and friendly contact' with workers which comes from 'a genuine and kindly interest' in their welfare. Furthermore, Fayol was keen on workers showing initiative which he saw as a source of strength for the organization. He planned to provide management education in schools (Parker and Ritson, 2005) and engage in management research by the 'sharing of observations, experiences … that would help all better understand this important matter of administration' (Wren et al., 2002: 910).

Stoney (2001) notes that the fundamental principles proposed by these early theorists continue to inform and influence the role and function of current management such as 'personal goal setting' within appraisals and 'management by objectives' both of which are common practice. Furthermore, the Taylorist 'one best way' is a clear antecedent of benchmarking, standardization, evidence-based practice and care pathways (Hewison and Griffiths, 2004). Both Fayol and Taylor used differential pay rates as motivators which are similar to modern pay bonuses, performance-related pay and profit-sharing for personal achievements (though not in healthcare).

The main critique of this system is its foundation on positivistic assumptions that science can be applied neutrally to human affairs, its perceived lack of concern for workers' autonomy and its inflexibility, relevant for 'modern' leaner, flatter and adaptable organizations.

Human relations theory

In contrast to the 'classical' approach, the human relations theory postulates that 'classical theory' is modified by people – their desire for social relationships, their response to group dynamics and their needs for personal fulfilment.

Amongst its proponents, Mary Follett, proposed a management system which deemed that improvements in productivity were due to social factors including a supportive style of management which:

- focuses on the work group whose motivation is satisfied by social and emotional needs and feelings of 'belonging';
- aims to improve effectiveness through valuing people as important organizational resources;
- facilitates achievements by focusing on building team spirit and commitment.

Mary Parker Follett (1868–1933)

Mary Parker Follett was a social worker and management thinker whose work, according to Salimath and Lemak (2005), has not been given sufficient attention partly because of her gender and the attitudes of the times in which she wrote and partly because of the difficulty in categorizing her work. She was also one of the first action researchers (McLarney and Rhyno, 1999) and therefore of particular interest in this text and her work is currently undergoing a radical reassessment as having significant contemporary relevance (Lemak, 2004).

Follett did not formulate a management theory but wrote a series of essays on leadership and conflict resolution (Fox and Urwick, 1973). Some of her ideas are incorporated into the model of management in Figure 4.1. Particularly she advocates:

- Participation – sharing power and responsibility of workers with managers using 'co-action' rather than 'coercion'.
- Management as facilitation – recognizing and valuing the various 'wills' of the group; working in teams rather than as individuals.
- The aim of the organization is to build and maintain dynamic and harmonious relations – groups not individuals are central.
- Group power comes from uniting under a common purpose – the goal.
- A true team works through the integration of individual differences.
- Conflict is positive and should be dealt with constructively through integration (see Chapter 10).

Follett is seen primarily through a management lens, but, through her ideas of integrating business, philosophy and life, she proposed a process of lifelong learning and, through that, the key to achieving lasting change (Salimath and Lemak, 2005). In the sphere of management, she advocates replacing the command and control style with a humanistic and negotiable approach 'that recognized and embraced complexity, flexibility, democracy and change' (Parker and Ritson, 2005: 1343–4).

Whereas Fayol stressed 'planning', Follett stresses 'co-ordination' particularly because:

- Everything is connected – a small change in one place has an effect in another; thinking should be 'un-departmentalized' (Fox and Urwick, 1973: 149).
- Early contact with staff while plans are forming will prevent future problems and better 'co-relations'.

- Through direct contact with people, differences can be resolved quickly.
- Co-ordination is a continuing process.

Finally, Follett stresses participation, seen as resting on understanding and co-ordination: 'Participation means two things; the contribution of each individual and the co-ordination of such contributions. For co-ordination we need understanding and for understanding we need openness and explicitness' (Fox and Urwick, 1973: 186).

An approach to managing

The above discussion indicates that management, as an area of study, is no different from psychology or sociology with many competing and conflicting theories, advocates and interpretations.

Many change management initiatives in healthcare are 'project' based and Figure 4.1 provides a model which illustrates some of the general 'planning' and 'people' management processes which are involved in such projects.

Though each situation is unique, there are general principles which can be applied in planning change events. Griffiths (DHSS, 1983: 11) stressed that what was lacking in healthcare was a 'clear management process' rather than the requirement to have a 'general manager' (Winyard, 2003).

Although the model (Figure 4.1) is depicted as sequential with a clear direction of travel and with two main sections emphasizing 'planning' and 'interpersonal processes', in practice the components are in a dynamic relationship with one another hence there is a constant need for monitoring, refining and feedback mechanisms. It further informs the change process in Chapter 6.

Main points of Figure 4.1

There is little doubt that developing and implementing effective change makes participatory team management a prerequisite for effective motivation and mobilization of human resources in organizations (Dervitsiotis, 2002). This requires sufficient capacity and opportunity for local flexibility and discretion in taking decisions and actions of how best to achieve aims as well as moving from a command and control environment to one of co-operation, sharing and mutual learning (see Box 4.1).

Pre-plan

A more detailed discussion of the factors influencing pre-planning can be found in Chapter 8, however, at this stage, the following points are noted:

- Planning processes begin with information collection (Burnes, 1996). The better quality information managers have, the better and more informed future decisions will be and in all organizations 'it is in the decision that everything comes together' (Goodwin, 1998: 28). Although evidence-based management is still rare (Walshe and Rundall, 2001), managers should ensure that actions are based on the best evidence available (Young, 2002).

External Health Policy Environment: Internal organizational, political and cultural climate →

Interpersonal processes and roles

Planning processes →

Communicate
– Vision/mission/rationale
– Plan – objectives & goals
– Philosophy & values
– Strategy & tactics
– Standards

Consult
– Work content & skill mix
– Negotiate responsibilities
– Delegate tasks & roles
– Listen, reflect & respond
– Facilitate participation & progress

Collaborate
– Teambuilding
– Team spirit
– Participation – ownership
– Support networks
– Organizational politics

Co-ordinate
– Lead → inspire
– Organize → control
– Educate → motivate
– Monitor & Appraise
– Problem solve

• learn
• re-plan
• pilot
• trouble shoot

A
C
T
I
O
N

• Achieve Solution
• Evaluate Results
• Lessons Learnt
• Develop Team
• Develop Individuals
• Develop Self

Pre-plan

Pre-Plan

Data
• gather
• receive
• sift
• sort →

Tools for analysis
SWOT
PEST

Stage 1

Strategy
Mission
Values
Quality
Culture
Power
Decision
Processes
Staff
Schedules
Milestones

Stage 2

Goals
Discuss, decide and agree →

Justify decision for
• task
• team
• time-frame
• self

Stage 3

Priorities
Discuss, decide and agree →

What
• must
• should
• could

be done by time limits and within budgets

Resources

Allocate:
• Human
• Financial
• Material
• Data
• Time
• Space

Monitor, reflect on and evaluate all activities and develop supportive networks and co-operative relationships →

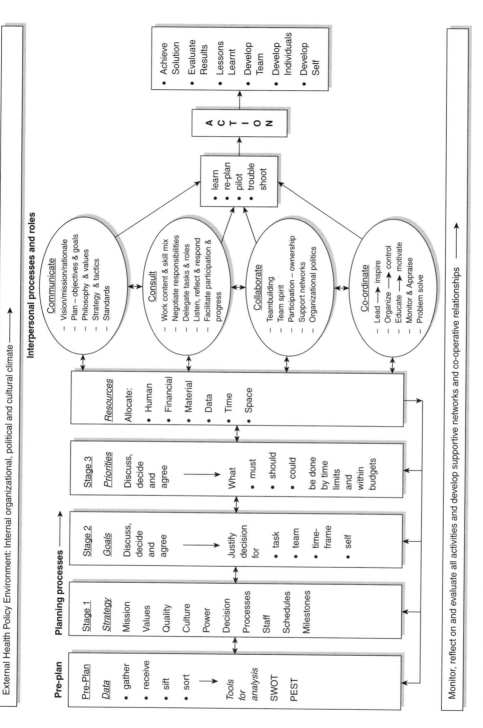

Figure 4.1   An approach to managing

Key data to examine revolve around contextual factors, including:

- Overall aims and mission of the organization.
- Priority of need for the planned change.
- Policy imperatives.
- Cost/benefit analyses.
- Extent of decision-making freedom.
- Finance and resource constraints.

- Johnson and Scholes (1989) suggest data are subjected to a SWOT analysis. This evaluation should enable managers to develop a 'perspective' (Mintzberg, 1994) to inform their strategy. Johnson and Scholes (1989) caution that information is dynamic and open to change, therefore opportunities and threats can change in the light of new data.
- In healthcare, the needs of the consumer/patient are the pre-eminent driving forces behind decisions (DH, 2000a, 2005; Guo and Anderson, 2005).

Planning

- Planning is one of the most important skills especially when dealing with a range of multi-professional staff and scarce resources.
- It is seen as time consuming and a diversion from seeing patients from a medical perspective but in service terms is the key to achieving better population health (Fitzsimmons and White, 1997).
- It involves setting and agreeing both long- and short-term goals, setting priorities, deciding on the optimum strategy for achievement and allocating resources.
- It diminishes resistance to change and, when staff are prepared, creates involvement and a sense of control (Fox and Urwick, 1973).

The Healthcare Commission's review of the quality of healthcare and public health in England and Wales notes that though waiting times have reduced, it believes 'less attention has been paid to ensuring that services are efficient or to planning for the long term' (Healthcare Commission, 2006: 97).

Strategy

- Goodwin (2006: 183) notes that there is little agreement on what constitutes a strategy. Furthermore, he claims that strategy and planning are interchangeable terms but that 'defining a strategy solely as a plan is insufficient'.
- Plans are basic statements of where the organization or group aims to be in some future configuration.
- Strategy details the means through which goals may be attained and related to the overall mission while encapsulating ideas about the organization's values and culture.
- Long-term plans have dubious value as political imperatives and policy changes occur so frequently. However, in shorter term projects, a purpose-centred 'road map' fosters motivation from team members and can prevent costly mistakes.
- Methods for measuring team performance and achievement should be set. Planning processes are evaluated in terms of their contribution to outcomes.

Goals

- Clear goal formulation is a key management role (Staniforth and West, 1995).
- Goals should be clearly stated, give purpose and direction to actions and be understood by participants. Wheeler and Grice (2000) suggest applying 'SMART' criteria (specific, measurable, achievable, relevant, timely).
- Participatory management implies goals are not imposed from above and staff are involved in goal setting. Where personal, team and organizational goals are congruent, effectiveness increases (Rushmer et al., 2004a).
- Bottom-up goals agreed and set by a team are more likely to be 'owned' and motivation and commitment to succeed will be higher (Sims and Lorenzi, 1992).
- Imposed goals may not be owned or understood by participants – motivation to succeed may be reduced.

Priorities

- Priorities focus on major needs of the service which should match the responsibilities, resources, skills and knowledge of the team.
- They should be realistic and include an awareness of the whole system and the impact of their cumulative load.
- They should be flexible in the light of changing circumstances and policy.

Resource allocation

- Plans must include a budget to achieve goals – this includes capital and revenue expenditures agreed with budget holders.
- Staff are an important resource and may need CPD requiring a training budget.
- There is a feedback loop from resources to all stages of the planning process to encourage continual monitoring and preparation of contingency measures.

Interpersonal processes

The concepts above highlight specific areas around the processes of planning in management. However, Goodwin (2006: 194) argues that when developing interdepartmental or organizational working it is individuals who do the actual business not the corporate management of services, therefore 'the development of sustainable interpersonal relationships is crucial to collaborative success'. These interpersonal processes are identified in the ovoids in Figure 4.1. Management approaches must balance the tasks and goals to be achieved with the means by which to achieve them. Traditional management in health services has been based on command and control systems and formulaic policy responses (Feldman and Khademian, 2001).

Communication, consultation, collaboration and co-ordination (Follett claims 'co-ordination is the most important point in organization; Fox and Urwick, 1973: 131) are the four key participative qualities of successful management (Parkin, 1998). They stress participative team management because 'executive line management is inappropriate in flexible, team based organizations where staff are educated professionals' (Thorne, 1997: 178).

As Michie and West conclude:

Studies across work sectors ... in healthcare consistently support the value of team-based working. This means developing team-based organizations in which education and communication systems, people management and reward systems and the culture are all geared towards managing teams rather than individuals. (Michie and West, 2004: 105)

Box 4.2 provides an example of the effectiveness of collaboration and teamwork in implementing management change which is developed further in Chapter 11.

Box 4.2

Overview

Cooper and Hewison (2002) report on a project to introduce a system of clinical audit into a palliative care setting. Palliative care is a relatively new discipline which has grown quickly in an unplanned way. Yet its ideals, structure and delivery are seen as embodying high quality practice creating a reluctance to embrace quality assurance methods, such as clinical audit, especially where practitioners have a high degree of autonomy. Following a review of audit tools, the Support Team Assessment Scale (STAS) was selected. The study followed an earlier attempt to implement an audit which failed because of the absence of a structured plan and insufficient preparation and training of staff.

Planning and data collection methods

1   A focus group was held with staff to discuss issues around the previous failed attempt. Participants were encouraged to express views and a SWOT analysis was used to structure the discussion and encourage greater collaboration.
2   Questionnaires were administered to assess staff readiness to implement STAS.
3   Five review meetings were held to discuss staff experiences of implementing audit and STAS.

Results and decision phase

Results showed that staff were concerned about:

• Ethical issues and the number of variables involved.
• Time commitment and the way data might be used.
• Lack of knowledge of STAS.
• The need for continuous clarification of details of the tool.

(Continued)

(Continued)

Implementation phase

- Participants collaborated on aspects of implementation including who should carry out the assessment, on which patients and how to reduce subjectivity.
- Limitations of the tool were identified around confidentiality, patient selection and time management.
- Implementation was facilitated via continuous co-operation, evaluation and feedback between participants and researcher.

Post-implementation group

This group met two months following completion and found that:

- Ownership of the change emerged as participants incorporated audit into their practice.
- Multi-disciplinary team working increased.
- Reflective practice improved.
- More positive attitudes towards audit emerged during implementation.
- Improvements in care were identified further increasing motivation.
- Levels of confidence improved as quality of practice was seen as the participants' responsibility.

Summary

This is a classic management situation where there is a need to collect data on clinical practice to inform the contracting process. Previous management driven change had failed through lack of involvement. Action research methods created a 'bottom-up' process of involvement, collaboration and ownership (see Figure 4.1) which prompted the staff's professional development, awareness of the research process and improved client care.

Clinical audit continues using a more comprehensive and refined STAS tool.

Contingency

In reality, plans become disrupted, priorities change and actions have a 'trouble-shooting' focus rather than a controlled sequence of carefully thought out performances. Innovation and adaptation are needed to produce an optimum service with limited or inadequate resources. This has led to the recognition of Follett's 'law of the situation' (Fox and Urwick, 1973: 29) where structures, processes and actions should be flexible and responsive to serious or sudden changes both from the external and internal environment.

The reality of managing may therefore be illustrated as Figure 4.2 rather than Figure 4.1. This does not mean that 'anything goes' – these dynamics and responses require managers

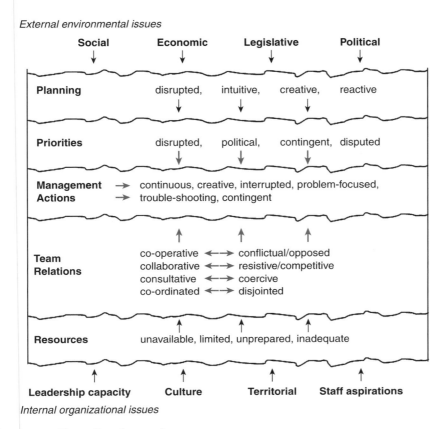

External environmental issues

Figure 4.2   The reality of managing

to make a careful examination to assess their impact and plan a response that best fits emerging issues.

Management and action research

Though they share many concepts, management and action research are not synonymous and the day-to-day management of a team or unit should not be confused with action research. However, where there are protracted practical problems for a workgroup in a local situation, action research offers a sound means of solution.

Altrichter et al. (2002) imply that when staff are keen to improve their work situations and are involved in gathering data, participation, power-sharing, collaboration, reflection and learning then there is the potential for an action research approach.

Whitehead (2005) also claims that project management shares similarities with action research. These include creating knowledge, solving problems and promoting change as well as using a knowledgeable researcher/manager who is immersed in the organization. Although he recognizes that there are differences, he advocates that using the principles of inclusion and participation from action research could ameliorate some of the weaknesses of project management and its rigid hierarchical processes.

Conclusion

Management theory demonstrates that when attempting to achieve goals and manage people in complex and dynamic situations there is no 'one best way' to handle tasks, manage change and solve problems in healthcare; there are no off-the-shelf recipes or solutions. Each staff group and local situation is different, with different policy drives, dynamics, needs and aspirations, and therefore strategies, plans and interpersonal processes are multifaceted and need to be contextually sensitive (Pettigrew et al., 1992) to achieve relevant outcomes.

In essence, the key to good management is open, honest communication and a clearly understood and updated strategy, together with participative implementation methods which value worker contributions.

Chapter summary

- Management theories rest on a continuum ranging from tight control to flexible participation.
- Management in healthcare has moved from consensus working to control through managerialism, emphasizing targets, protocols, performance measurements and evidence-based decision making.
- Managerial work emphasizes actions of planning, priority setting and budgeting.
- Healthcare management should emphasize communication, consultation, collaboration and co-ordination.

5

Leadership in Healthcare

Introduction

The key to implementing successful change in healthcare is leadership integrated with effective management processes.

Leadership research, anecdote and opinion has created a vast and bewildering range of literature (Hunt, 1992) characterized by a myriad of competing terms and definitions; theories and models; qualities, actions and skills; as well as historical shifts in fashions (Michie and West, 2004). The lack of consensus over meaning can be seen by claims that there are more than 1,500 definitions of leadership (Gill, 2006) and more than 65 classification systems (Northouse, 2004).

Furthermore, leadership has been examined from a wide range of disciplines, particularly business and psychology, each of which has focused on and studied its favourite constructs, creating its own set of categories and theories (Gill, 2006). Constructs can encapsulate the essence of leadership theory within one discipline and yet be ignored by another. This fragmentation has lead to weaknesses in the scope, scale and maturity of leadership theory which remains devoid of any accepted criteria or parameters (Kakabadse, 2000). Furthermore, the creation of constructs originating from business studies may lack application to healthcare. There are few randomized control studies and these are often unsuccessful, therefore data tend to be generated mainly from less robust observational studies (Naylor, 2006).

Recurring themes within leadership literature include debates on differences between leadership and management; whether leaders are born or made; the lists of roles, styles and traits of leaders; leadership as an exclusively executive function; the place of leadership ethics; and the role of the context in creating conditions which enable leaders to emerge. Contextual features refer to an organization's mission, culture and structure, the opportunities and threats of the market, the environment and the position of the organizational life-cycle. Young, dynamic and smaller entrepreneurial and commercial organizations will require different leadership from older, larger, bureaucratic public-sector organizations.

These variations have been difficult to control within empirical studies. However, consistent research has shown that the popular 'trait and characteristics' school where a single individual in a leadership position can have a comprehensive overview of an organization's finer details and can harness and motivate its resources to successfully achieve goals, is flawed and unsustainable in today's complex world (Degeling and Carr, 2004; Hewison and Griffiths, 2004). Furthermore, no set of personality characteristics has been found to occur consistently in leaders. Indeed, the reverse is more likely to be true – historically leaders are noted for being different from each other (Hunt, 1992; Avery, 2004). It is clear that there is no single or simple model which can apply in all situations (Hewison and Griffiths, 2004).

More recently in healthcare, theorists have concentrated in separating 'transformational' leadership, termed 'flavour of the month' (Degeling and Carr, 2004: 402) from 'transactional' leadership where faith is firmly placed with the former, seen as the saviour of the healthcare system and the only option to effect the significant change required for its future survival (Trofino, 1995; DH, 1999; Outhwaite, 2003; Millward and Bryan, 2005; Murphy, 2005). But just as transformational leadership is being developed in the NHS (Alimo-Metcalfe and Lawler, 2001), in the post-modern era, even this convincing but simplistic dichotomy is seen as outdated (Van Wart, 2003).

It is not the purpose of this chapter to rehearse these aspects and it is beyond its scope to analyse the numerous theories and models of leadership. It therefore aims to:

- outline the relevance of leadership to managing change in healthcare organizations;
- discuss the main definitional issues;
- discuss the key differences between management and leadership. This is pertinent since governments in the UK (DH, 2000a), America (Trofino, 1995) and Canada (Davis, 1997) promote the move, in language terms at least, from 'managing' to 'leading' in healthcare;
- outline the core processes of leadership derived from research which can be learnt and developed in individuals;
- consider current research on leadership in healthcare practitioners, teams and organizations.

Leadership and change

Initiating and managing change in groups, teams or organizations of whatever size causes fundamental disruption to systems, structures and plans, and, more significantly, causes pain and discomfort to people – particularly the organization's staff, but also the initiators and managers of change themselves. Understanding, communicating and managing these disruptions requires thought, planning and attention to the organization's mission, culture and value systems. This warrants the involvement of people with particular skills at every step from initial idea and design to completion and evaluation.

The importance of effective leadership is not disputed. As Van Wart asserts:

In organizations *effective* leadership provides higher-quality and more efficient goods and services ... a sense of cohesiveness, personal development, and higher levels of satisfaction among those conducting the work ... an overarching sense of direction and vision, an alignment with the environment, a healthy mechanism for innovation and creativity, and a resource for invigorating the organizational culture. (Van Wart, 2003: 214)

In times of disruption, however, the means of achieving these conditions are compromised. Those with leadership skills need to clearly prepare the ground through communicating their own or the corporate vision, build confidence and consensus through support and explanations concerning the inevitable uncertainties and questions, and prepare the ground for future consequences and difficulties – in other words, help followers make sense of the change. In healthcare, these actions, and the opportunity to carry them out, are often compromised through the politicization of health; the remoteness of the policy-making forums; the multitude of professional bureaucracies (Berwick et al., 2003); the lack of a single constituency (and non-participation of many constituents); and the lack of a 'corporate' identity. For innovations in healthcare to be sustained these structural challenges require a broader, more inclusive view of leadership than has hitherto been the case.

Analysing terminology

Appleyard (2002) claims that leadership is the most ambivalent and hypnotic of human qualities but that it also has strange, elusive and enigmatic characteristics which, despite the best efforts and observations, are still far from being understood (Appleyard, 2005). He explains that people recognize leadership qualities when they encounter them but find it difficult to separate and describe, let alone analyse, what those qualities are. This 'normative' quality is recognized by Van Wart (2003) when he refers to the nineteenth-century, and still popular, theory of the 'great man' and its counterparts 'hero' and 'genius' – to which now might be added 'entrepreneur' and 'celebrity' – and their ability to move and shape attitudes and affect the paths of progress. A modern example of the latter may be peripherally known pop stars or comedians mobilizing politicians, governments and populations worldwide to 'feed the world' and 'make poverty history'. However popular these figures may be, because of the rarefied nature and scarcity of examples in society, Van Wart claims they are unusable in any scientific theory. The 'great man' theory perpetuates the common myth that there exists an exceptional, omnipotent person who can solve all organizational problems single-handedly (Avery, 2004). It also implies that leadership cannot be developed through training and experience or by being the right person in the right place at the right time with the right audience (Westley and Mintzberg, 1989). Peck (2006: 326) states that the 'great man and trait' theories are 'alive and kicking' in healthcare settings, particularly amongst politicians. This leads to the re-cycling of successful 'leaders' to failing organizations in the mistaken belief that success will follow them from one situation to another.

Gill (2006) raises the conundrum of 'good' and 'bad' leaders where language unhelpfully fails to distinguish between 'good' meaning leaders who are morally good or 'good' meaning effective. Morally bad leaders may be effective (in terms of achieving goals and motivating followers) but can they be described as 'good leaders'? This depends on the views of the 'followers' who ascribe leader status, though it may be untenable to describe ineffective leaders as 'good' simply from a moral position. This is seen, for example, in politics where leadership is so valued that people agree that someone is a 'good leader' though they may disagree with or disapprove of their ideals.

Alimo-Metcalfe and Lawler (2001: 392–3) present a useful typology:

1 'Rational-legal' leaders who achieve their organizational position, such as Chief Executive Officers and senior managers, through merit having demonstrated they have the knowledge, skills and abilities to function at that level. Their 'leadership' derives from their formal authority (Hartley and Hinksman, 2003).
2 'Charismatic' leaders who may not occupy the top organizational positions as the rational-legal leader but who, through their personality, ideas and rhetorical skills, connect with the needs of followers. Such individuals may be found in politics, sport and the media.
3 'Traditional' leaders where power is based on the office held and to which deference and respect is shown because of that office; positions include the monarchy and high religious or public office.

These distinctions are not new. Writing in 1928 about the leadership role of industrial nurses, Follett uses the terms 'leadership of function, personality and position' respectively (Fox and Urwick, 1973: 282). She predicted that the 'leadership of function' which describes those with knowledge and skills to control situations, would become more important in successful organizations.

An interpretive complication arises with the 'functional' leader when individuals are assigned to positions where 'leader' is part of the job title, as in 'clinical' or 'team' leaders. This frequently occurs in healthcare but the role, decision making powers and scope for 'leadership' actions are severely curtailed by internal factors such as organizational and professional culture, territorial and line management issues and prescriptive procedures as well as external factors such as economical, legal and political restrictions. Opportunities for innovation can be thwarted by centralized authority and the chain of command (Brazier, 2005) which diminishes and nullifies the notion of leadership. Bureaucracies are subject to powerful forces beyond leaders' control which can make their contributions relatively insignificant (Van Wart, 2003). These individuals are termed 'formal' leaders and this allows for the recognition and potential for 'informal' leaders to emerge and lead on different initiatives by using expertise (Rushmer et al., 2004a: 401). Indeed Follett recognizes the significance of different degrees of leadership capacity and that 'different situations require different kinds of knowledge' and, where individuals possess that expertise, they should be enabled 'to become the leader at that moment' (Fox and Urwick, 1973: 281).

Rushmer et al. (2004a) further differentiate 'hard' leadership which is about providing structure and systems to 'make things happen' from 'softer' leadership which focuses on caring and supporting interests around the needs and concerns of others to build capacity and confidence.

Leadership and management

Chapter 4 stated that the term management was derived from the Latin *manus*, the hand, and hence to the term 'to handle' a thing or situation. In relation to leading, Gill (2006: 8) claims that it is derived from the Old English *lædan* meaning to 'take with' or to 'show the way' (Schwartz, 1988). This indicates that leadership is not necessarily concerned with external control mechanisms through co-ordination and delegation but functions at the more emotional level of inspiration and education to create internal motivations. Generally management systems are devised to control and give direction, whereas leadership draws and motivates followers through development (Bruhn, 2004), though in practice there is significant overlapping of skills, processes, activities and the means of achievement. The terms are frequently used interchangeably in the literature. This conceptual conflation can be seen in Lord Laming's admonishment of managers in a situation of abject failure in the running of public services:

> What is needed are managers with a clear set of values about the role of public services ... combined with the ability to 'lead from the front'. Good administrative procedures are essential to facilitate efficient work, but they are not sufficient on their own and cannot replace effective management.
>
> This Inquiry saw too many examples of those in senior positions attempting to justify their work in terms of bureaucratic activity, rather than in outcomes for people. (Laming, 2003: 5)

The conflation is entirely appropriate where 'rational-legal' managers (Alimo-Metcalfe and Lawler, 2001) are required to demonstrate leadership skills. Hunt (1992: 248) concludes that 'the major difference between managing and leading is the leader's capacity to lift people up, articulate purpose, give reality to higher values and resolve conflicting aims as a means to the fulfillment of the followers'. Greenwood (1997: 22) links leadership to change and claims that 'a manager is someone who maintains a person, situation or group. A leader is someone who moves that person, situation or group, that is, brings about change'. In these examples, 'managing' is seen as a relatively constant position whereas 'demonstrating leadership' can be temporary depending on the people involved, the needs and dynamics of the context, and the relative capacity of the actors.

Management and leadership are not synonymous but neither are they mutually exclusive, rather leadership can be seen as a sub-set of management (Albritton and Shaughnessy, 1990) (see Figure 4.1). A restrictive conceptual dichotomy is found in McKenna and colleagues' study (2004: 73) where community nurse responders state that 'nurses are often encouraged to be managers rather than leaders'.

Leaders therefore are called to be inspirational, whereas to be an effective manager does not necessarily require inspiration (Hunt, 1992). If leadership is seen as emotional, conceptual and intellectual then it need not be related to position, status or authority roles within an organization and can be dispersed more widely than is commonly assumed. Management is position based, leadership does not have to be.

Transformational and transactional leadership

Burns (1978) argues that most leadership theory can be seen as 'transactional'. This tends to represent a mechanistic, bureaucratic approach focusing on specific rules, policies and procedures for handling predictable matters (Brazier, 2005) and the operational, day-to-day aspects of daily work. Transactional leaders are oriented towards means within a prescribed role (Kakabadse, 2000). This has been called 'management by exception' either with an active component where managers closely monitor work and take action to correct mistakes, or passively where sanctions are imposed after mistakes have been made (Northouse, 2004). Transactional leadership derives from 'exchange theory' and is used to refer to a barter or transaction from leaders to subordinates which promotes better performance by offering tangible and extrinsic 'contingent' rewards, usually money, recognition and promotion, or sanctions. This forms around a power-based relationship as it is in the self interests of subordinates not to cross the demands or preferences of their leader. According to some definitions, this may not be leadership at all but may best describe contemporary operational management with the transactional leader resembling the traditional manager (Murphy, 2005). It works within the status quo and existing structures, so change tends to be incremental and focuses on symptoms (Ferlie and Shortell, 2001).

In contrast, transformational leadership refers to inspiration and intellectual stimulation (Keller, 1995) and 'lifting the motivational and moral cohesion of the group such that the common weal dominates over rational self-interest' (Hunt, 1992: 258).

The fundamental task of leaders is to 'bring into consciousness their followers' sense of their own goals, values and purpose'. Leaders therefore elicit meaning for what followers want to do. By this process, they 'make the followers more conscious of aspects of their identity – function, profession, background … and give that identity relevance' (Hunt, 1992: 248). Effective leadership therefore is an interaction between individuals and their context (Hartley and Hinksman, 2003).

Any changes implemented by transactional leaders are termed 'first order' or 'single loop' – of process or procedure (Argyris and Schon, 1978). Transformational leaders make 'second order' or 'double loop' changes which would have a lasting benefit because they changed systems, perspectives and ways of thinking. Transformational leaders influence through motivation by appealing to basic values (liberty, justice, altruism and achievement) and through being a catalyst for change, hence they can disrupt the status quo and replace it with a new order. Transformational leaders, Van Wart (2003) claims, understand a changing environment, facilitate more dramatic changes and energize followers more than transactional theory suggests. Criticisms of these claims abound, however, particularly in their perpetuation of leadership as a characteristic trait (Northouse, 2004), and lack of conceptual clarity (Yukl, 2006). In healthcare, transformational dimensions and contingent reward have been found to ameliorate exhaustion in healthcare workers whereas leaders who continuously monitor performance and intervene to correct mistakes generally increase levels of stress (Stordeur et al., 2001).

Core leadership concepts

In an attempt to synthesize the main concepts from 50 years of research, Northouse (2004: 2–3) argues that leadership is much more complex than might be assumed. The major concepts suggest that leadership can be seen as:

- The product of group processes which includes power relationships between the leader and followers.
- A combination of situations and characteristics creating a 'personality perspective'.
- Actions or behaviour focusing on creating change in individuals and situations.
- Instrumental in helping people achieve goals.
- Having a set of particular skills.

From these concepts Northouse (2004: 3) concludes that leadership is:

- a process;
- involves influence;
- occurs within a group;
- involves goal attainment.

Similarly, Hunt (1992) claims leadership is the capacity to mobilize a potential need in a follower. It is a relationship or process of mutual stimulation and elevation that converts an arousal of need into engagement, action and results. Leaders have the ability to raise consciousness and awareness (of values, needs, aspirations and purpose) within followers thereby giving meaning to possibilities. Leadership therefore enhances voluntary compliance to an idea through influence (Bass, 1990; Greenwood, 1997).

By seeing leadership as a process or interaction between people rather than a characteristic indicates that leading is not linear but dynamic, interactive and available to all (Northouse, 2004).

Yukl (2006) believes that the leadership role is about inspiring, developing and empowering followers. It is not about authority, administration, control or supervision. It is concerned with 'exercising influence' (Thorne, 1997: 171) over others to help them understand and see what needs to be done and how it can be done effectively through the process of facilitation. Northouse distils this further: 'Leadership involves influence: it is concerned with how the leader affects followers. Influence is the sine qua non of leadership. Without influence, leadership does not exist' (Northouse, 2004: 3).

Gill (2006) states that five common themes seem to capture the essence of individual leadership:

- Vision and a sense of mission or purposefulness.
- Creating a culture of positive shared values (termed 'consideration').
- Developing and implementing strategies for the pursuit of vision and mission (termed 'initiating structure').
- Empowering people to be *able* to do what needs to be done.
- Motivating and inspiring people to *want* to do what needs to be done.

Within these major themes, Burns (1978), Bass (1990), Kotter (1990), Hunt (1992), Kakabadse (2000), Hartley and Hinksman (2003) and Yukl (2006) argue that, at the individual level, there is some congruence on how to describe leadership. Ferlie and Shortell (2001: 290) use the term 'portfolio of leadership approaches' whereas Hartley and Hinksman (2003: 7) state it is 'a set of processes or dynamics'. These approaches avoid creating specific, innate skills and characteristics, combine management and leadership concepts, generate the conditions and opportunities for change and align with the three key areas on which leaders generally focus: the individual, group and task (Adair, 2004):

Cognitive	Information management – competent marshalling of facts, figures and ideas (see 'pre-plan' stage in Figure 4.1); concept formation and concept flexibility – assessing and developing ideas into potential changes; weighing up of possibilities to create a vision and developing strategies for its achievement; 'framing' – conceptualizing and defining purpose and values into reality.
Interpersonal	Enables participation through consultation with others (see 'consult' in Figure 4.1); manages interactive skills which enhance people's abilities; shares influence; develops orientation to plans and visions through coaching, training and feedback; builds teams through consensus; works with a wide range of people; effectively uses coalitions; displays integrity.
Presentational	Ability and personal confidence to communicate visions clearly and articulately (see 'communicate' in Figure 4.1); ability to scan an audience, anticipate problems, take risks and build trust; pro-active orientation to mobilize resources; impression management; presenting, articulating and transmitting task and organizational values through intellectual stimulation.
Self-awareness	Takes responsibility for initiating; displays confidence and networking skills; demonstrates pro-action to achieve plans; recognizes and develops skills and abilities in others; shows emotional maturity; demonstrates self knowledge and self regulation; acknowledges weaknesses (Naylor, 2006).
Value-congruence	Understands the organization's guiding principles and the needs and aspirations of staff and customers; achievement-oriented; sets standards for others to follow and aspire to (termed the 'management of meaning', Yukl, 2006: 272).
Vision	Develops orientation, aims and essential values for progress towards vision and improvement and defines methods for achievement; coaches, trains and motivates, creates an 'achievement orientation'.

Vision is seen as the essential quality of being able to envisage the future state to which the organization aspires and needs to move towards (Alimo-Metcalfe, 1996). Westley and Mintzberg (1989: 17–18) break this down into three distinct stages:

1   envisioning an image of a desired future organizational state which, when
2   effectively articulated and communicated to followers serves to
3   empower those followers so that they can enact the vision.

Westley and Mintzberg (1989: 19–20) link vision with presentation and articulation skills as in Churchill's 'we will fight them on the beaches', Martin Luther King's 'I have a dream' and Shakespeare's Henry V 'we band of brothers' speeches. They argue that visionary leadership works through skilled use of rhetorical devices and that '*how* the vision is communicated becomes as important as *what* is communicated'.

They see visionary leadership as a dynamic, interactive phenomenon as opposed to a unidirectional process but also argue that strategic vision must take into consideration strategic content as well as the strategic contexts of the product, market, process and organization, thereby integrating leadership with management.

Critique of leadership concepts

These core competencies are claimed to contain the main forms of awareness that underlie leadership: intellectual or cognitive; emotional; spiritual; and behavioural (Gill, 2006). There are cautions, however. Firstly, never will any one person be skilled in all areas. Ancona et al. (2007) argue that it is time to appreciate the importance of 'incomplete' leaders who recognize where their strengths and weaknesses lie and appreciate the need to work with others who have complementary leadership skills.

Secondly, leadership qualities are frequently promoted with hyperbole and applied uncritically, particularly within nursing literature, using similar literature as endorsement but with scant regard to empirical evidence (Jooste, 2004). Jooste asserts:

> There is a special bond between nurses that cuts across language, culture, specialist knowledge and practice circumstances that allows us to share with one another our art, skill and wisdom. The time has come for leaders in nursing to shape nursing practices that changes in society, politics and healthcare services demand. Nursing must do this before other professions dictate what the nursing role in healthcare organizations will be. (Jooste, 2004: 222)

These comments take little account of the powerful political, structural and cultural forces within organizations which can thwart even the most well organized group (Parkin, 1997).

Finally, leadership competencies focus on the individual and thereby perpetuate the 'great man' myth or, in Georgiades and Phillimore's terms, the 'myth of the hero-innovator' described as

> The idea that you can produce, by training, a knight in shining armour who, loins girded with the new technology and beliefs, will assault his organizational fortress and institute changes both in himself and others at a stroke. Such a view is ingenuous. The fact of the matter is that organizations, such as schools and hospitals, will, like dragons, eat hero-innovators for breakfast. (Georgiades and Phillimore, 1975: 315)

Other writers add that in order to be successful in making structural changes, leaders must have the authority to act or sanction the actions of others (Rushmer et al., 2004a: 401). Degeling and Carr (2004) call this 'institutionally grounded' – leaders do not have free rein and actions are always circumscribed by what is authorized by the institution.

Leadership in healthcare

At the macro level, the *Capability Review* of the Department of Health (Cabinet Office, 2007: 18) criticizes its leadership in not setting out a 'single clear articulation of the way forward'. Since staff lack clear direction, they feel disenfranchised and little sense of ownership of any vision leading to 'a limited sense of working together to achieve a collective purpose'.

At the clinical level, the arguments and conflicts between medicine and management set out in Chapter 4 are similarly rehearsed within the reforming agenda of leadership. Degeling and Carr (2004) reassert the structural pre-eminence of medicine as having legislative and ideological backing for its monopoly position in the labour market, which is continually reinforced through clinical and policy encounters. Thorne (1997: 171) argues that a working definition of clinical directors suggests they are primarily change agents and shapers of meaning who influence others to follow a desired course of action. While agreeing that doctors should in theory be the natural leaders in healthcare since they are industrious, ambitious and articulate, Naylor (2006) and McHugh et al. (2007) argue that they are often poorly equipped since training favours individual achievements rather than consensus building and they lack sufficient emotional intelligence. This individualism has cemented the 'consultant as leader' belief through references to 'my patients, my registrar and my beds' (Treasure, 2001: 1263). Doctors who become consultants in acute specialities, who are traditionally seen as leaders in hospitals, tend to be goal driven, analytical and less compromising in their style (Treasure, 2001). Other commentators point to observational studies which reveal the defects in communication between doctors and other clinical staff (Olsen and Neale, 2005). This can be seen in instances such as the review into the Oxford Cardiac Services (National Health Service Executive (NHSE), 2000) which found a serious lack of leadership, surgeons working autonomously, a culture of complacency and secrecy leading to difficulties in recruitment and retention of staff and a decline in service quality (Dobson, 2000). The report noted that 'there appears to be a lack of common vision, with each surgeon functioning as an individual unit, some with little regard for the others' (NHSE, 2000: para 3.2).

Writing about his views on leadership, Appleyard draws from Adair's theory (Adair, 2004) and concludes that between 1 in 10 and 1 in 15 nurses has leadership potential. Appleyard (2005: 4) says that if 40,000 of the 350,000 nurses could be turned into leaders, 'our second most hopeless public service after the police would be galvanized'. The NHS Plan appears to provide opportunities to support this. Box 5.1 illustrates a study designed to develop potential healthcare leaders.

Box 5.1

Overview

Kelly et al. (2002) report on a one-year funded study designed to establish and develop a new, supernumerary clinical practice facilitator's (CPF) role in six pilot sites in a large inner city teaching hospital. The role aimed to support newly registered nurses (RN) and healthcare assistants to enhance their competence and clinical skills. The project's objectives were to pilot, evaluate and identify the potential of the role, determine key factors contributing to success, and develop a framework for practice.

CPFs were expected to help junior staff develop clinical skills, provide leadership and teaching and facilitate support and supervision for individual staff.

Action research was the chosen method as it promoted collaboration and reflection and enhanced participants' confidence.

Exploratory and planning phase

The transition from student to RN is stressful and newly qualified RNs require support from experienced colleagues to develop their competence and knowledge.

Baseline data were collected through:

1   Ward Organizational Features Scale (Adams et al., 1995 cited in Kelly et al., 2002) sent to all nursing staff. Relevant categories included: staff organization; professional practice, ward teaching and learning; practice development and job satisfaction.
2   Recruitment and retention data.
3   Assessment of educational audits.

Results from the exploratory phase:

- Low response from questionnaires, however, 80 per cent of managers felt that junior staff were encouraged to develop new skills and knowledge compared to only 18 per cent of RNs who felt they were supported to reach their potential.
- Staffing levels – over-reliance on agency staff.
- Lack of time for clinical supervision.
- Lack of suitable feedback on performance.
- Lack of support for new ideas.
- Low staff morale.
- Lack of support for professional development.

Decision and action phase

CPFs were recruited to six sites. Support in the new leadership roles was maintained through monthly meetings, notes were recorded and circulated, and researchers visited pilot sites. CPFs responded to exploratory data via clinical teaching sessions, managing poor performance, developing effective relationships with managers, balancing expectations of the role with the organizational restraints, developing teaching skills and accessing staff to development courses. CPFs developed a profile across the Trust and

(Continued)

(Continued)

maintained reflective accounts of their actions. The reflective accounts, feedback and meetings enabled a framework for CPF practice to be developed.

Evaluation phase

Eighty per cent of CPFs who had been in post for eight months or more returned questionnaires. Ninety-five per cent stated they were satisfied or highly satisfied with the new role. Staff generally found them approachable, motivational, beneficial and supportive to junior staff.

CPFs themselves evaluated their new role as working with staff to plan change and provide support through the process. The role was enhanced through not being 'managerial', being less threatening to managers and a bridge to roles in practice development and education. The CPF role was perceived as a valuable resource within the Trust.

One participant evaluated the experience in an MSc dissertation and found that the facilitation process included fostering clinical leadership, establishing boundaries and control, enhancing knowledge and skills and promoting a transformational culture.

Summary

The study shows how action research enabled a small group of select staff to become a team of leaders and initiate and develop leadership roles proving beneficial to less experienced colleagues and the wider organization. This has occurred through leadership actions, teaching and facilitation skills. The CPFs were supported through the process and enhanced their skills, practice and value to the organization.

From management to leadership in healthcare?

The language of the *NHS Plan* (DH, 2000a: 86–7) changed from the historical policy focus on management to the 'modern' focus on leadership (Learmonth, 2005): 'Delivering the plan's radical change will require first class leaders at all levels of the NHS'. Yet the example cited where ward sisters will be 'given authority to resolve clinical issues such as discharge delays and environmental problems such as poor cleanliness' (DH, 2000a: 86) and 'draw up local clinical and referral protocols' (DH, 2000a: 86) fall under the umbrella of operational management in terms of control, supervision and everyday problem solving rather than the rhetoric of transformational leadership discussed above. This supports Hartley and Hinkson's (2003) contention that basic practices are relabelled as 'leadership' to suit the organizational rhetoric. Appleyard graphically depicts the difference:

> Management is now a dirty word – it reeks of sacking people with fancy excuses about de-layering and right-sizing. Leadership, however, has a warm, human ring, suggesting collective effort and comradeship – managers are desk bound cowards, leaders are heroes, scaling the heights. (Appleyard, 2002: 28).

This 'heroic' language began with *Making a Difference*:

We need visionary leadership to help build modern, dependable services and to inspire and sustain the commitment of nurses, midwives and health visitors during a period of significant change. Strong nursing, midwifery and health visiting leadership is needed at every level. It is needed to drive forward interagency and multidisciplinary team working, to improve quality and practice through clinical governance, to lead public health initiatives, to plan and commission services locally through Primary Care Groups and Trusts, and to provide effective management of clinical services and corporate functions. We need to develop the leadership skills of more nurses, midwives and health visitors to meet this challenge. Our plans to improve health and healthcare call for a particular style of leadership. We need nurse, midwife and health visitor leaders who can establish direction and purpose, inspire, motivate and empower teams around common goals and produce real improvements in clinical practice, quality and services. We need leaders who are motivated, self aware, socially skilled, and able to work together with others across professional and organizational boundaries. (DH, 1999: 52)

This is aspirational in the extreme. However, the strength of professional cultures in healthcare (see Chapter 7) and the rigidity of bureaucracies (see Chapter 8) means that in their desire to reform, leaders find little room for manoeuvre and cannot stray far from the organization's protocols, or from the values and beliefs of clinical staff, most notably doctors who are most resistant to reforms (Degeling and Carr, 2004; Greener, 2006). Despite the superlative claims from the Department of Health (1999) above, Degeling and Carr (2004: 406–9) found nurse leaders 'at the bottom of a system under pressure' and particularly stressed and lacking in power. Furthermore, they found medical clinicians regarded nurses as having only limited authority on clinical practice issues, which they saw as rightfully located in the medical domain. General managers too felt 'sandwiched' between the reforms promoted by the policy makers and hospital senior management and the resistance of medical clinicians. In reality, managers are involved in 'managing the disjunctions in the system' rather than displaying a real leadership role as defined above.

Everyone's a leader?

In its desire to create a patient-led NHS the UK government notes: 'Cultural change of the order required will take time. Success will depend on every single member of the NHS demonstrating leadership in promoting the values and vision of the NHS' (DH, 2005: 26).

In his discussion on leadership, Kakabadse (2000) uses examples of tribal warfare in primitive societies. All warriors were expected to perform heroic acts in warfare and hence, through their acts, all were heroes; but, since all were heroes, the lack of 'exceptional' actions made them all ordinary so there were no heroes at all even though they undertook heroic acts. Kakabadse shows that the real leaders were the tribal elders, labouring in the background, not being heroic or transformational, but working towards peace through negotiation, exchange, bargaining, and 'transactions'. Kakabadse illustrates that what is required is both transformational and transactional leadership and that the different skills provide for different needs which emerge from different contexts, tasks and people – Follett's 'law of the situation' (Fox and Urwick, 1973: 29).

Primary care

In primary care it is claimed that:

> Nursing will need effective leadership if it is to take on new roles, work differently and deliver the improvements for patients and communities. This requires greater understanding of team development and the management capability to use human and financial resources creatively and effectively. (DH, 2002c: 10)

The reality may be rather different, as shown by McKenna et al. (2004). They examined attitudes of general practitioners, community nurses, policy makers and the general public regarding nursing leadership in primary care. Findings from general practitioners and nurses support the default view that the doctor (and budget holder) is the 'rational-legal' leader (Alimo-Metcalfe and Lawler, 2001), therefore the 'natural' leader of the team. This fits with Goodwin's (1998: 30) assertion that 'those who occupy positions of centrality' and 'exercise control over information' are most likely to emerge as leaders. Further findings indicate the general confusion around leadership in community nursing and the belief that nurses with leadership qualities leave practice or are moved into management (McKenna et al., 2004). Similarly Rushmer et al. (2004a) claim that the power of the general practitioner, as an independent practitioner running a small business, cannot be underestimated as a strong influence on what other practice staff are able to achieve.

Williamson (2005) reports an action research study designed to promote work-based learning and to evaluate and strengthen the implementation of shared governance and identify factors that facilitate or prevent effective decision-making by clinical leaders. The study followed members on three practice-based councils charged with implementing shared governance across a health Trust. Though claims are made that leadership was enhanced, results showed that members felt ill equipped and under-prepared for the role. There was frequent misunderstanding of the role and remit of the councils and a lack of a 'Trust-wide' view. The use of a framework to organize meetings was reinforced as beneficial but rarely used resulting in meetings which were disorganized. Whereas great attempts were made to empower clinical leaders in their roles as council members, the actions were far from those specified by the Department of Health policy above (DH, 1999).

In health visiting, Hyett (2003) argues that health visitors are denying their leadership role by clinging on to their independent ways of working. Hyett claims that in times of reduced staffing and extra work, moving to more co-operative, team-based approaches will promote shared goals, common objectives and more time spent on planning with the primary healthcare team.

Reviewing the evidence of leadership development in nursing, particularly the Leading Empowered Organizations (LEO) programme (Miller, 2000), Hewison and Griffiths (2004) found that following training participants delegated more, improved their communication skills and planned ahead more, but few were able to identify a specific example of the impact of the course on their clinical care. Rather, the courses were popular as they provided the opportunity to be absent from work and to 'network' in a multidisciplinary environment. In a survey of 5,000 staff in the NHS, local government and the private sector Alimo-Metcalfe and Alban-Metcalfe (2003: 29) found NHS leaders scored lowest on the items of 'inspiring others, supporting a developmental culture, encouraging change, being honest and consistent, acting with integrity and showing genuine concern'. The last item was found to be 'the single most important indicator of transformational leadership' but was among the weakest dimension in NHS leaders. Furthermore, managers were found to 'hold back morale by lacking inspiration and failing to support change'.

The study found most senior managers relied on 'status' as evidence that they 'had what it took to be leaders' so did not need 'development'. Furthermore, they believed their junior staff needed training but they failed to respond to their ideas once they returned from courses – suggestions were 'rejected or ignored by their defensive bosses' (Alimo-Metcalfe and Alban-Metcalfe, 2003: 31) mirroring the exploratory phase results in Box 5.1.

Leaders of teams or teams of leaders

Following Smith's (2003a) charge concerning the NHS as 'not having a leader' raised in Chapter 1, there followed an email conversation between three influential discussants (Berwick et al., 2003: 1421) where one of the discussants, Ham, argues that the NHS needs 'lots of leaders at all levels and not just a single leader'. Ham claims that collective leadership or 'coalitions' will be more effective in uniting the top-down and bottom-up approaches. This means that there needs to be more organizational members with 'discretionary' rather than 'prescriptive' powers for decision making. Berwick defined this as a 'team at the top' with a balance of leadership skills who engage in dialogue, respect and interaction. This echoes claims by Staniforth and West (1995) that the concept of 'distributed' leadership should be considered, however, they caution that teams of leaders can suffer from unclear goals, slow decision making, role conflict and negative synergy, where synergy is defined as 'the whole being greater than the sum of the parts' (Staniforth and West, 1995: 28). Previous claims by consultants of 'my patients and my beds, etc.' must be replaced by 'our service, our team, and our role' (Treasure, 2001: 1264). Regarding the Oxford Cardiac Services, the report strongly recommends that the five surgeons:

> Must function as a team with a common vision of the way forward … This means an ethos of trust…combined with a friendly attitude of 'give and take'. If the consultants cannot sign up to this type of code of practice, they should seriously consider their future. (NHSE, 2000: para 7.1)

Belbin (1981) has long described the model team as comprising eight or nine key roles. Although his classification has been criticized for lack of evidence, it has had an important impact in the UK (Fisher et al., 2000). The roles are categorized respectively as:

- 'person-centred' – extrovert, with tendencies to stability (roles include: co-ordinator/chairman, team worker, implementer, resource-investigator). These are good at forging relationships, communicating and supporting people.
- 'task-centred' – more introvert and anxious (roles include: the shaper, plant, monitor-evaluator, completer-finisher) and more individualistic. They specialize in creating and challenging ideas and engage in forensic examination and evaluation.

Fisher et al. (2000) argue that people-oriented roles consistently produced higher levels of participation, work interest and effectiveness. Belbin (1981) and Fisher et al. (1998: 286; 2001: 580–1) suggest that the two opposing 'leadership' roles of 'coordinator' and 'shaper' are complementary and counterbalancing – the former unifying the team and the latter driving it. Fisher et al. (1998) concluded that a balance of 'person' and 'task' focus were unlikely to be found in the same person indicating that a mixed set of roles in leadership is optimal (Reay et al., 2003). In their later study of nearly 1,800 male and female managers in the UK, Fisher et al. (2000) found a surfeit of co-ordinators and resource investigators suggesting that some organizational teams may be unbalanced. There is no extrapolation of these data to healthcare, however Millward and Bryan (2005) argue that the role of 'clinical leader' is clearly one of managing relationships, interpersonal dynamics and the communication process which can be observed from the example in Box 5.2.

Box 5.2

Overview

Reid et al. (2007) report on an evaluation of the implementation and impact of an 18-month pilot project in the UK for the assessment and rehabilitation of older people with complex needs. The service introduced three interdisciplinary Rehabilitation Link Teams (RLTs) drawn from health, social and voluntary agencies which provide clients with intensive rehabilitation, co-ordinated and delivered through multi-agency collaboration. Action research was used to promote learning and change through regular feedback in order that emerging issues could be addressed during the 'bedding in' of the new service.

Exploratory phase

1   Data to evaluate the implementation of the model were collected through:
- (i)   36 days observing the work of the RLT members' activities and interactions;
- (ii)   six focus groups each with managers and support workers regarding team-work issues, quality of service and cross-boundary work;
- (iii) interviews with 3 RLT managers on two occasions;
- (iv)   two-phase postal surveys with stakeholders including nurses, GPs, social workers, volunteers (n=105).

---

2   Data to evaluate the extent that the model enabled independent living were collected through:
    (i)   36 interviews with clients and carers;
    (ii) outcome measurement on 73 clients over 12 months.
3   To evaluate the impact of action research on RLT members a half day workshop was used

Emerging issues from data

Two examples of emerging issues are raised here:

Issue 1:

- At 7 months, focus groups revealed that team members were concerned that their 'care-manager' role lacked clarity, they were unable to make full use of their uni-professional clinical skills, they felt unprepared for their role and vulnerable and anxious when faced with hostility from interagency partners.
- Acute sector responders complained that referral criteria to RLTs were too restrictive causing inadequate response and discharge delays, and that role duplication would confuse clients.

Response phase

- Monies were obtained to run a series of interagency workshops to explain and clarify new roles.
- A communication strategy for wider team members and partner organizations was established.
- A re-appraisal of referral criteria occurred and a flow-chart developed to illustrate the access process.
- Profession-specific competencies were developed for each care manager occupation group (district nurse, social worker, occupational therapist).

Issue 2:

At 16 months, data from the focus group with homecare workers raised concerns regarding: lack of role clarity; inadequate 'rehabilitation' activity and responsibility; hostility from mainstream homecare colleagues who did not understand their position in the new scheme; difficulties with contracts and confusion over managerial lines of control.

Response phase

- Recognition by team managers that the issues were important.
- Work delegation and managerial structures clarified.
- Managers' understanding helped overcome the barriers and progressed the change project.

(Continued)

(Continued)

Overall response to action research

Responses were overwhelmingly positive, particularly concerning the ability to enable timely accounts of experiences, reflection on work, and transformative thinking regarding barriers that had to be overcome to enable change to occur. The range of data used enabled a holistic understanding and distribution of organizational knowledge and the development of a collaborative culture.

Summary

The study shows that successful change can be enacted through using a whole systems approach which enables individuals, groups and organizations to learn, adapt and improve continuously. A prerequisite for this situation is a transformational leader who has a clear vision, exemplifies the values and beliefs of the mission and has a 'whole-system approach to change' (Reid et al., 2007: 63).

Conclusion

Throughout this chapter it has been asserted that the modernist 'great man' theory of the single charismatic leader, developed from Nietzsche's conception of 'superman' so beloved of politicians and the head-hunter industry is outdated and a mistake (Kakabadse, 2000; Ferlie and Shortell, 2001). Leading healthcare has to diversify to value the notion of horizontal and distributed leadership and display flexibility in developing and achieving plans and a compendium of approaches which enable that most tantalizing of skills – crossing occupational, cultural and territorial boundaries with equanimity – to emerge.

Chapter summary

- The rhetoric of implementing health policy has moved from a focus on 'management' to championing 'leadership'.
- The idea of organizations having a single leader is outdated.
- Leadership should be seen as a set of processes or approaches which can be learnt and applied in different contexts.
- Leadership ability is widely dispersed within an organization.
- For the effective implementation of change in healthcare, both management and leadership approaches are required.

6

Approaches to Change

Introduction

Chapters 1 and 3 have set the current context and imperative of change in the health policy arena and the wider world, Chapter 2 promotes action research as a viable, pragmatic and attractive method for implementing change and Chapters 4 and 5 raise the importance of cultivating management and leadership approaches to assist in planning and implementing change initiatives. They are necessary but not sufficient to enable healthcare practitioners with the confidence to implement improvements in their workplace as required under current health policies.

Organizational change in healthcare is one of the hardest objectives to achieve since there is an assumption that implementation will be unproblematic (Saka, 2003; Diefenbach, 2007) and the application of a linear and rational approach (Ashford et al., 1999; Lamb and Cox, 1999: 292) will be successful. The complexities and challenges of change however are legion; Huczynski and Buchanan (2001) claim its triggers, directions and consequences are a highly complex blend of human, social, cultural, political, economic and technical processes that have yet to be systematically understood. Yet McWilliam and Ward-Griffin (2006) argue that if any group has the mandate and potential to lead change initiatives which improve human conditions and optimize potential, then it is those working in health and social services. Despite this view, many writers note that change efforts are fraught with difficulties (Parkin, 1997; Salauroo and Burnes, 1998; Macfarlane et al., 2002), fail (Ferlie and Shortell, 2001) or suffer from 'initiative decay' where any gains are lost through the eventual abandoning of new practices (Buchanan et al., 2005). For example, at the macro, strategic level, Winyard (2003: 468) points to the Kings Fund evaluation of the internal market, arguably the deepest change ever wrought in the UK health service, which found that though it fundamentally altered attitudes to the funding and delivery of healthcare, it made little discernable difference to its actual delivery (Le Grand et al., 1998). More recently, the planned implementation of the Medical Training and Application Service (MTAS) originated by the NHS Plan to manage junior doctor's jobs, has systematically failed to achieve its aim (Shannon, 2007).

At the, operational level, McMurray and Williams (2004: 352) report on a survey in a large public health institution in Australia examining the extent to which nurse managers' styles, perceptions and knowledge of their organizational structures are factors impacting on their ability to be innovative in their workplace. In answer to a question identifying areas where they felt they were 'innovative at work', out of 82 potential responders only two managers believed they were innovative and had the insight, skills and instincts to be successful in managing change. They report that despite moving from a dictatorial structure to more decentralized management that is supportive of innovation, negative comments such as 'why bother' indicate that decision processes were manipulated at unit level and innovatory ideas were blocked by business managers. Massey and Williams (2006) report on the 'CANDO' system of workplace organization in an NHS Trust in the UK; the four change agents experienced problems with staff attitudes and believed that managers blocked change as they thought they were doing a good job and the proposed changes were not needed, despite the project being supported by senior management. These examples demonstrate not only the wider organizational and structural difficulties of implementing change, but also the human, motivational and psychological challenges, particularly where operational management has been devolved to practitioner levels. Though initiatives provide renewed vigour at their inception, the visionary period often loses momentum and may eventually expire (Buchanan et al., 2005). Jarrett (2003) claims that 70 per cent of change management programmes fail and Orgland (1997), who summarizes change research throughout the 1990s, notes that the main barriers to successful change are employees' lack of implementation skills and their undermining of, and resistance to, change efforts. The studies above also point to managers themselves preventing change.

This chapter aims to examine the change process by discussing a range of issues which need to be reflected on and engaged in to work towards effective change management. If healthcare practitioners are to gain confidence in dealing with and implementing change then sound knowledge of change theories, methods and processes are essential (Balfour and Clarke, 2001). These include:

- defining change – meanings, metaphors and models;
- knowledge required to initiate change;
- factors affecting the change process;
- proposal of a model of change;
- the role of action research in implementing change.

Parkin brings these themes together in identifying the complexity of the change process:

> Charisma, communication skills and a good idea are not enough to be successful at implementing change. There are certain qualities and skills required that integrate notions of power and status; leadership, motivation and tenacity; high levels of communication, empathy and conflict management; characteristics of foresight, creativity, and planning as well as knowledge of research, evaluation and politics, and the obligatory practice of questioning the habitual and familiar … Managing change is difficult and messy … fraught with problems and is often unsuccessful or at best, short-lived. (Parkin, 1997: 133–4)

These comments integrate some key aspects of change implementation, specifically management and leadership, and the content and context of the change idea, which are developed in the chapter's emerging model of change. Although potential opportunities to implement change which are within the sphere of healthcare practitioners' influence are shown in Table 1.1, Dunphy (1996: 541) cautions that there is no single, all-embracing and widely accepted change theory and no agreed guidelines for action by change agents.

Change – meanings, metaphors and models

Meanings

The term 'change' is value-neutral and should be differentiated from ideas of progress, improvement and development, which, while still suggesting something different, indicate a positive trajectory. Bertrand Russell (1950) states that whether any change has occurred is scientific and irrefutable, but to describe a change as 'progress' invites an ethical and political debate depending on the perspective of the observers and participants. For example, the term 'climate change' is value-neutral, whereas 'global warming', discussed in Chapter 3, indicates a certain philosophical and political positioning which has already made judgements about particular data. Handy (1993) argues that change is a necessary condition for survival and, in organizations and individuals, is a never-ending search for improvement to gain competitive advantage – to simply maintain the status quo in the current climate is not an acceptable option. Indeed, in the perpetually fast-moving environment of modern society 'not to change is to lose' (Parkin, 1997: 139).

Current health policy favours the term 'innovation' to indicate something 'new' combined with positive progress. The *NHS Plan* (DH, 2000a: 56) states that devolving power to frontline staff will give 'the chance for health professionals to innovate locally, earning greater autonomy the better they perform'. This seemed to have been achieved when, four years later, the *NHS Improvement Plan* (DH, 2004a: 11) stated that 'A new spirit of innovation has emerged, centred on improving the personal experience of patients as individuals, and this is now taking root in the NHS'. Much of the literature on change management, however, points to it being unpopular and causing stress, conflict and unexpected problems (Stewart and O'Donnell, 2007). The term 'innovation' may appear softer since, as Pryjmachuk (1996) notes, while change may be unwelcome, 'innovations' rarely are.

Theorists use a collection of terms to define change including 'strategic', 'transformational', 'organizational', 'fundamental', 'incremental' and 'second order'. There is clearly a difference between strategic change (concerned with strategy, structures, systems and leadership, Buchanan and Badham, 1999: 61) and incremental change (concerned with operational issues) but Weick and Quinn (1999: 375) note that many small adjustments, created across a number of entities accumulate to create substantial change. For analytical purposes two generic types are discussed: episodic and continuous.

Metaphors

It is unsurprising that metaphors derived from nature and horticulture abound in change management theory. *Delivering the NHS Plan* (DH, 2002a: 5) mentions the NHS 'growing organically' and the claim that innovations are 'taking root' (DH, 2004a) has already been noted. Handy (1993: 292) questions whether change can be 'managed' at all, rather he suggests that to 'cultivate change' is something different, suggesting an attitude of growth, of challenging rather than controlling, learning rather than instruction – a changing organization is one 'that uses differences to grow better'. Johnson (1998) alludes to the tidal 'ebb and flow' of the changing environment and of seeing organizational development as the flowing of a stream. Paton and McCalman (2000: 9), however, argue that organizations should not be seen to be 'merely bobbing about on a turbulent sea of change' and that they can make proper choices to control their strategic positions and manipulate their environment in order to achieve their ends. The horticultural metaphor of growth and renewal implies a natural, evolutionary and cyclical process of change and this theme is taken up by Weick and Quinn (1999) who highlight the contradictions inherent in defining change. They argue that recent analyses of organizational change suggests that there is an important distinction between change that is 'episodic, discontinuous and intermittent' and change that follows the 'growth' or life-cycle metaphor which is 'continuous, evolving and incremental' (Weick and Quinn 1999: 362). As Pryjmachuk argues (1996: 202) 'change is, to some extent, the very essence of life'. These differences in the perception of change are important and have significant impact on the models used to describe and analyse it and the attitudes and methods with which it is approached.

Episodic change

Weick and Quinn (1999: 366) see episodic change as occurring at distinct periods of an organization's life cycle. This may occur at the macro level, perhaps precipitated by triggers such as new technology, knowledge or legislation; the introduction of new personnel, such as a manager or chief executive with new ideas and plans; external threats such as changes in availability of materials or skills and product obsolescence; and internal threats such as workforce changes or general inertia. In this view, change is infrequent (termed 'punctuated equilibrium' – a series of one-off instances within longer periods of stability, Jarrett, 2003: 25) and intentional and is often created in the wake of the perceived failure of the organization to adapt to its environment. Orgland (1997: 6–7), describes it as 'an alteration between long periods when stable infrastructures permit only incremental adaptations and brief periods of revolutionary upheaval'. These periods of upheaval produce fundamental change which occurs in 'short bursts of simultaneous changes in many variables'.

Continuous change

In contrast to episodic change, Weick and Quinn (1999: 366) define continuous or emergent change as a constant and evolving state. Thus change is 'a pattern of endless modifications in work processes' carried out at the local and micro level and a 'continuous process of adaptation to flux in the environment' (Hartley et al., 1997: 61). Change is a continuous cyclical process without a pre-determined end state and therefore change tends to have a longer term perspective and emphasizes a learning process. As Parkin states:

> An alternative perspective views change in organizations, and indeed society as a whole, as an inescapable and continuous process, a never-ending journey of discovery, development, growth and realignment with the environment; and as a process of constantly creating ideas to achieve individual and organizational potential while responding to external pressures in order to maintain viability. (Parkin, 1999a: 21)

As with all generic types these views are reductionist and socially constructed by theorists. It is more instructive to conceive them as points along a continuum along which the reality of practice, and life, fluctuates.

Models of implementation

There are numerous models and theories of change which have been developed over the last 60 years which often, conceptually, distinguish between 'linear' and 'circular' approaches (Orgland, 1997). However Hendry (1996) and Burnes (1996, 2004) claim that most accounts of organizational change implicitly follow the three-step model developed by Lewin (1947/1997: 313–24) of 'unfreezing, change of level, and freezing on the new level' (in his brief description of 'changing as three steps', Lewin does not use the term 'refreeze'). Despite its ubiquity in the literature, and his brief account, it forms only part of his overall theory of social change which includes action research, field theory and group dynamics (Burnes, 2004). Burnes (1996) shows that other writers have added to Lewin's basic three-step model but he argues that it remains recognizable in all planned approaches to change. Burnes expresses his concern about change models that are too prescriptive and argues that the planned approach is coming under increasing criticism.

Planned approaches   SPT

The planned approach to change is the method of implementation most commonly associated with episodic change. The process is seen as a deliberate and conscious attempt at changing a situation usually involving an agent, often a manager, and a system, which may be a work group, team or organization. The focus is often to apply new knowledge, skills or technology to practice, in order to modify systems, behaviour and attitudes and to improve overall performance or productivity (Brooten et al., 1978; Bennis and Nanus, 1985). It treats an organization as a machine where specific inputs are made to create certain outputs.

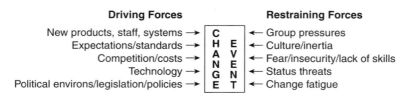

Figure 6.1 A force field

Source: after Lewin (1947/1997: 313–24), Coch and French (1947).

This approach recognizes that groups and organizations usually exist in a state of equilibrium. This balance is seen by Lewin as being maintained by two sets of forces – the forces driving towards movement and change and the forces which attempt to maintain the status quo through resistance (see Figure 6.1).

Lewin (1946/1997: 351) claimed that the restraining forces did not lead to change ('locomotion'), rather they influence the effect of the driving forces. This could be something as simple as an individual's lack of skills or knowledge but strong forces for change will inevitably produce strong counter-measures to maintain balance. Planned interventions tend to be imposed from the top down, are structured, organized, goal-orientated and linear and may be facilitated by external forces (see Table 6.1).

Interventions usually aim to produce anxiety, discomfort but psychological safety in workers and have a beginning and an envisioned end point. Implementation tends to cause disruption through the disconfirmation of the current position.

There is evidence that managers tend to rely on linear models of diffusion (see Figure 6.2) despite their lack of empirical validity (Fitzgerald et al., 2002). They are also seen as increasingly inappropriate with too much reliance on managers preventing freedom of choice for participants (Saka, 2003).

The planned approach is exemplified by two examples. Firstly, Sir John Harvey-Jones who, following his visit to a UK Health Authority and witnessing managers' disastrous

Table 6.1   Dimensions of change management approaches

Mechanistic approach	Dynamic approach
Making or creating a formula	'How-to' formulas redundant
Application of routine procedure/blueprint	Creative/experimental approach
Single method implementation	Shared/multiple implementation methods
Linear progress	Cyclical/spiral progress
Produces resistance	Resistance diffused
Single power source	Multiple/shared/collaborating sources
Authoritarian style	Participative/democratic style
Culture ignored	Culture/subcultures recognized
Product target	Process journey
Passive learning	Active learning

Source: adapted from Parkin (1999a) with permission of the *British Journal of Community Nursing*.

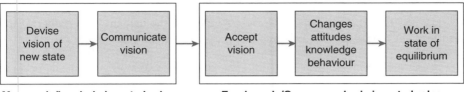

Manager's/Leader's imputed roles   Employee's/Group member's imputed roles

Figure 6.2 Theoretical model of linear, planned change for stable, non-problematic environments

Source: adapted from Parkin (1999a) with permission of the *British Journal of Community Nursing.*

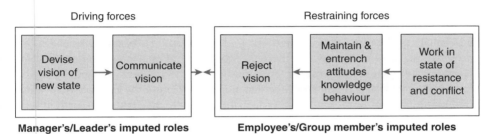

Manager's/Leader's imputed roles   Employee's/Group member's imputed roles

Figure 6.3 Possible reality of planned change for stable, non-problematic environments

Source: adapted from Parkin (1999a) with permission of the *British Journal of Community Nursing.*

attempts to close four hospitals, claimed that managers saw their role as being to 'formulate plans in isolation and, thanks to their breathtaking logic … expect everyone to go along with them' (1990: 147). This approach works, he claimed, if the proposed change is uncontroversial and there is consensus over the problem and the means of solving it but breaks down as soon as something more radical is required. Secondly, Salauroo and Burnes (1998: 460) studied the movement from institutional to community-based mental health and the closure of a large mental health institution. They noted that the view of the ineffective manager charged with implementing the change was 'that once the objectives were set and timescales agreed, everything else would run like clockwork'. In fact the attempts at the closures resulted, in both examples, in uncertainty, conflict and demoralized staff. The reality of the 'mechanistic' approach may be closer to that shown in Figure 6.3.

Paton and McCalman are clear about its weaknesses:

> The difficulty is that most organizations view the concept of change as a highly programmed process which takes place as its starting point the problem that needs to be rectified, breaks it down into constituent parts, analyses possible alternatives, selects the preferred option, and applies this relentlessly – problem recognition, diagnosis and resolution. (Paton and McCalman, 2000: 8)

This Taylorist, mechanical characteristic of the industrial age is seen as a 'flawed response' to contemporary problems (Johnson, 1998) and that 'encouraging participation means that a mechanistic, authoritarian and "top-down" approach is no longer viable' (Parkin, 1999a: 26). Bamford and Forrester (2003) argue that the uncertainty of the environment renders planned change inappropriate and an emergent approach more pertinent.

Emergent approaches

Emergent approaches to change appreciate the uncertainties of modern organizations. They recognize the rapidity and complexity of changes in the environment that make it impossible to envision and decide on a predetermined end point. Since change is seen as a constant state, approaches are less dependent on producing detailed plans and projections, rather they focus on 'reaching an understanding of the complexity of the issues and identifying the range of possible options' (Bamford and Forrester, 2003: 548). This encourages a 'bottom-up' process where the workforce takes greater responsibility for identifying problems and working on solutions in the manner implied by action research (see Table 6.1). Plsek and Greenhalgh (2001: 627) use the example of termites building a hill – they point out that these constructions are the highest on earth in relation to the size of the builders yet there is no chief executive, no architect and no plans. The termites act and work locally with others and, following simple shared behaviours and communication, the hill emerges from a process of self-organization. Orgland (1997) argues that when people see change as a continuous process, their behaviours become more proactive, involving experimentation, risk-taking, problem-solving and knowledge transfer leading to more successful and enduring outcomes. Change therefore has no beginning or end (Weick and Quinn, 1999).

Levels of change

Change can be analysed as occurring at different levels. Kumar and Thibodeaux (1990) propose an 'escalation' approach depending on the level of significance:

- First level – improving unit or departmental effectiveness.
- Second level – introducing change at organizational sub-systems level.
- Third level – organization-wide shifts in values and ways of working.

Parkin (1997, 1999a) has also suggested a three-level approach (Table 6.2) identifying the *macro* level as the influence of wider political, policy and institutional systems raised in Chapter 3, the *meso* level which considers organizations, professional groups and changes in management and leadership, discussed in Chapters 4, 5 and 7, and the *micro* level focusing at the personal interactive level discussed in Chapters 9, 10 and 11.

Ferlie and Shortell (2001) suggest four levels of change adding an 'individual' level, though Lewin (1947/1997: 329) argues that change targeted at the individual level is much weaker and that 'it was easier to change individuals formed into a group than to change any one of them separately'.

Table 6.2   Levels and units for analysing change

Levels of Change Events	Units of Analysis
Macro level	Social/political/legal systems Economic policies Environmental issues Globalization Cultural beliefs Health policies Demography Education policies Health care professions
Meso level	Organizations, Institutions, Health Trusts Employment practices Management styles Corporate missions Contractual obligations Professional Groups Health Centres/Clinics, GPs' surgeries
Micro level	Individual practitioners' interactions, meanings and perceptions Managers'/leaders' styles Teamwork/leadership skills Team's/group's aims and objectives Inter-professional interactions Professional role beliefs and values

Source: adapted from Parkin (1999a) with permission of the *British Journal of Community Nursing*.

Proposal of a change management model

Fitzgerald et al. (2002) argue that collectively studies show the diffusion process as being highly complex and critically influenced by a number of contextual characteristics. In the public sector, particularly in healthcare, there are specific dynamics requiring any approach to be contextually sensitive (Pettigrew et al., 1992). Methods for analysing the organizational context are discussed further in Chapter 8. Plsek and Greenhalgh argue that to cope with the escalating complexity in healthcare, linear models should be abandoned and replaced with 'New conceptual frameworks that incorporate a dynamic, emergent, creative, and intuitive view of the world ... [and] accept unpredictability, respect (and utilise) autonomy and creativity, and respond flexibly to emerging patterns and opportunities' (Plsek and Greenhalgh, 2001: 625, 628).

The change model in Figure 6.4 applies an emergent process to change management, proposes an integration of key aspects of the action research process (see Chapter 2 and Figure 6.5) and uses a range of influencing factors seen as most pertinent within health-care situations. A/R has been shown to

Specifically this approach recognizes the complexity of the change process through the identified 'influencing factors' on the left hand side. In its 'process approach' on the right, it promotes an iterative and dynamic approach to innovation and problem-solving

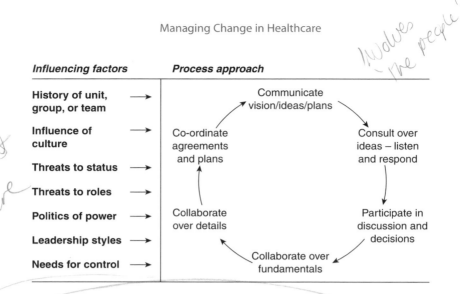

Involves the people (handwritten)

Figure 6.4   Dynamic model of managing change

Source: Parkin (1999a) with permission of the *British Journal of Community Nursing*.

(Jarrett, 2003: 26) which reflects action research through the interpersonal processes and roles of communication, consultation, collaboration and co-ordination which are transposed from the 'approach to managing' in Chapter 4, Figure 4.1. Furthermore, by including 'participation' within the cycle it offers a means of ameliorating resistance and further replicates the processes and philosophy of action research. Although it is not always possible to gain complete agreement on aspects of the change process, the cycle within the 'process approach' works towards achieving participation and unity in goals which are highly desirable conditions for successful change (Saka, 2003). However, as can be seen from the research examples provided in the text, the dynamic process means the end result cannot be predicted. As Koeck (1998: 1268) asserts, 'changing organizations is a process that will involve a series of learning cycles; this makes long range planning futile and demands a continuous reassessment of changes and intermediate results'. It therefore enables continual reflection and reaction to events, policies, priorities and personnel.

Factors influencing the change process

The influencing factors identified in Figure 6.4 have been developed through an examination of the literature on change management and, though they are not exhaustive, are the most significant in affecting the change process. Through the set of influencing factors, the model recognizes that effectiveness will be 'situationally determined' (Ferlie and Shortell, 2001: 283) by both the specific and wider dynamics of the organizational and political environment. It is therefore proposed that change practitioners need to be aware of and handle these factors which are now discussed. Pettigrew et al. (1992) suggest that change is a dynamic interaction between the context, process, and the content of change though the context in which problems exist is often ignored in traditional, linear models of change (Hall, 2006; Jarrett, 2003).

History of unit, group or team

An organization's or group's culture (see Chapter 7) is influenced by its history and maturity which produces 'organizational memories' (Bamford and Forrester, 2003: 560) and affect change initiatives. An organization's history is derived from:

- The people who have worked in it, their stories, achievements, failures and conflicts (see Chapter 10).
- The heroes, demons, geniuses and other characters who have worked together, their relationships, likes and dislikes.
- Previous attempts at implementing change and the residual feelings and perceptions resulting from them, particularly if these imply 'we've seen and heard it all before'.
- The journey taken together which collectively contributes to the creation of values, experiences and cultural practices.
- Attitudes to the work and social environment such as space, proximity, leisure time and socializing opportunities which influence communication patterns and affect the development of interpersonal relationships.

Outhwaite (2003) proposes that a leader's essential skill is to understand this history of service visions, values and goals and, in so doing, appreciate the rationale behind change and the feelings of fear and anxiety which may be generated. In Currie's study (1998: 21) of a culture change programme of management development in a hospital trust which used an industrial model of planned change, participants were simplistically advised to 'act as teams, to accept group responsibility and to disregard their historical individualism and professional isolation' thus creating covert and overt resistance and conflict. Managers in the study felt that the context in which they worked and their professional background had little empathy with the concepts of managerialism being implemented. History therefore implicitly links employees' learning with the ability of the organization to learn and hence to change (Johnson, 1998). The strength of a group's history can often be felt when new employees join and are seen as a disturbing influence:

> [Newcomers] … do not take the wisdom of our ways for granted. They therefore ask questions which we do not know how to answer, because in the past we had no occasion and saw no reason to ask them ourselves: 'Why do you do it this way? Does it make sense? Have you tried it differently?' The way we have lived, the kind of life which gives us our security and makes us feel comfortable, is now challenged. It has turned into a matter we are called to argue about, explain, justify. It is not self-evident and does not seem secure anymore. (Bauman, 1990: 59)

In the grip of change, individuals and groups have to move from the familiar to a less well-defined future; they need to leave behind their comfortable habits and behaviours and be exposed to developing new skills, knowledge and attitudes and this is fearful for them and difficult for the manager (Mintzberg, 1994). Plsek and Wilson (2001) argue that good practice spreads more quickly where leaders respect the patterns of past efforts to innovate.

Influence of culture

The influence of professional and organizational culture on change efforts is explored in more detail in Chapter 7 but here the significant influence of organizational culture within the change process as a system of social control is raised. Johnson (1993: 61) argues that the reality for any organizational action is hedged and protected by a web of cultural artefacts – symbols, myths and rituals which legitimize the organizational constructs and routines and 'programme the way ... members respond to given situations'. Professional culture also finds its expression in learned, shared and inherited values and in the beliefs, norms and practices of groups. Importantly these values are seen to guide processes of thinking, decision-making and behaviour implying that change practitioners should recognize and account for the strength of cultural values and facilitate groups in their re-creation.

Ferlie and Shortell (2001: 294) suggest that a group-oriented culture 'emphasising affiliation, teamwork, co-ordination and participation' is associated with greater implementation of quality-improvement practices in contrast to a hierarchical culture focusing on rules and regulatory relationships which is negatively associated with successful implementation. Box 6.1 shows an example of a multi-professional approach geared to service improvement.

Box 6.1

Overview

Seymour and Davies (2002) report on their five-year involvement in the planning for child abuse investigation and therapy and in the development of Child Advocacy Centres in New Zealand.

Background

Their work indicated that there were deficiencies in the processes for investigation, treatment and litigation related to child abuse cases.

First exploratory phase

Their first fact-finding stage was talking to frontline practitioners to ascertain impressions. Davies met with social workers, psychologists, doctors, police and crown prosecutors

---

(later extended to administrators and judges in the Family and Criminal Courts) and discovered strong interest in improving services.

Decision and action

A group including all the above, additional representatives from minority Maori and Pacific Island groups and two mothers of children involved with the service, was set up to define the extent of the problem and design the research.

Second exploratory phase

1   Interviews held with 124 parents and 51 children regarding their experiences of child sexual abuse investigation, treatment and litigation processes.
2   Transcripts of court proceedings were examined.

Findings

Several major deficiencies were revealed:

- Delays in service provision.
- Poor service co-ordination leading to contradictory advice.
- Poor uptake of therapy services.
- Inadequate support for non-offending parents throughout the process.

Decision and action

Findings disseminated; training provided for all professional groups involved; conference presentations and local publicity raised the profile and interest in changing the service.

Third exploratory phase

Development of new model of service delivery – 'child advocacy centres' combining services of police, child protection, medical examinations and prosecution in one building.

Decision and action

Plans for a 'centre' submitted to state services at Wellington; building of multi-agency centre comprising police, evidential video unit, psychological and social work unit and medical team; lobbying government and judiciary led to funding for an 'education-for-courts' pilot programme.

Summary

Over the previous 10 years, services had become disjointed and antagonistic to each other. The action research process created new ways of co-operating and a shared sense of purpose. Work continues to develop the multi-agency model.

Although Burnes (1996) does not refer to healthcare specifically, he notes that organizations that have a 'role' culture align better to planned change because of its 'top-down' model of management. He argues that it is difficult to see how such an organization could adopt the decentralized and participative approach of the emergent model. Similarly, Weick and Quinn (1999) argue that using these methods in large organizations is counterintuitive since size and participation are often negatively associated.

Threats to status

Davis (1997: iii) asserts that the roots of dissimilarities among healthcare workers stem from differences in education and training, professional socialization, psychological orientation, diverse knowledge, values and cultures, and different ways of perceiving the world.

Olsen and Neale (2005) claim that attempts at collaboration can be undermined by differential power and status and lack of inter-professional socialization.

Ferlie and Shortell (2001) report that some innovations experience mixed acceptance due to incomplete participation by physicians and their lack of information sharing and communication with managers. In healthcare, there are ongoing debates about whether change initiatives should be management, medicine or nurse led (Massey and Williams, 2006) but an ideal implementation model is one where information is shared with participants and status differences are reduced.

Threats to roles

Workers feel safe, comfortable and confident in their habitual roles that they have nurtured over time. Implementing change threatens this comfort bringing 'loss of absolutes that characterise a previous, less uncertain time' (Davis, 1997: iii). When roles are subjected to change they can result in the loss of valued symbols, structures and relationships that had previously served as clear demarcations of someone's responsibilities. Macfarlane et al. (2002) report on a 'Community Based Medical Education in North Thames (CeMENT)' project organized between three large London medical schools which aimed to increase the amount of community-based teaching to medical students. They report difficulties and tensions concerning lack of clarity of aims, boundaries, roles and responsibilities and problems with leadership. At its heart were questions over ownership of the project, decision-making responsibilities, what the main focus of the research was, tensions over the curriculum, lack of mutual respect between GPs and hospital specialists and disagreements over methods of evaluation. Though the project was successful from a teaching perspective, it caused a 'substantial human cost' in terms of the stress experienced (Macfarlane et al., 2002: 321). A factor in this stress was the multiple roles played by clinical lecturers who also acted as trainers, co-ordinators, researchers and clinicians. The multiple roles led to 'role overload, role uncertainty and role conflict … from divided loyalties between the medical school and the CeMENT project' (Macfarlane et al., 2002: 322).

Because of its bottom-up approach, action research re-orientates power to practitioners. Where there is a high degree of centralized intervention and command and control this can militate against an enhanced role for managers and practitioners (Currie, 2000). However, reporting on an action research project to introduce an innovative Nurse Practitioner role into a GP practice in the UK, Livesey and Challender (2002: 173) report that the practice nurses already in employment felt marginalized, were intensely hostile to the researcher as they saw her as the 'instrument of their destruction' and were therefore 'difficult to engage ... in any meaningful discussion about how the new role ought to be developed'. Role change needs perceptive management.

Politics of power

Coghlan (2007) notes that any form of action or research in an organization has political dynamics and that political forces can undermine, subvert and block change efforts. When organizations are in a state of change and where the balance of power is modified or upset, political activity will intensify (Nadler, 1993). This may involve subverting plans, finding ways around organizational or group agreements or constraints, denying access to key data or personnel or even lobbying for the removal of personnel (Hendry, 1996).

Buchanan and Badham (1999: 231) argue that the change agent who is not politically skilled will fail. Harvey-Jones (1990) asserts that all managers must develop political skills which he sees as dealing with people, exerting influence, motivating and cajoling them into action and using conflict creatively to bring about change. However Saka (2003) reports internal change agents idealize a rational decision-making process which becomes detached from politics claiming their reasons are their continual confrontation with politicking in practice. Professional groups can engage in 'defensive boundary inhibiting behaviour' (Massey and Williams, 2006: 671) which creates friction and thwarts negotiation efforts. In their study, the change agents report dealing with staff from other departments as problematic. In their action research study to introduce a ward-based self-medication programme, Balfour and Clarke (2001) report initially that pharmacy staff used their expert knowledge to establish a power base to give medication advice, and at times both pharmacy staff and nurses experienced tension in their ability to 'let go' of the practice. The researchers claim that 'power issues' over-rode all other factors though eventually patients were 'allowed' to retain control over their medications.

Sharing power can also be threatening to leaders where empowering others may diminish their own power base. Where goals and methods are open to choice, they can be contested (Hartley et al., 1997). Change practitioners therefore need to be secure about their leadership role and self-confident in relinquishing power.

Leadership styles

Leaders have considerable influence over the 'climate' (attitudes and feelings) of situations which can affect performance and group satisfaction (Gil et al., 2005). Studies report that the 'we-feeling' which tends to decrease group members' aggression is diminished where there is autocratic leadership (Lewin, 1947/1997: 315). Change practitioners therefore need to be able to understand and empathize with the emotional impact and strain that any change programme brings and this is critical as a procurer of 'ownership' (Massey and Williams, 2006).

Change exposes the complex relationships between organizations, leaders and staff and the need to establish a high level of trust is vital for personnel to be encouraged to engage in risk-taking (Stewart and O'Donnell, 2007). In the CeMENT project discussed above, tensions arose between those leaders who initiated the project and those responsible for implementing and managing it. Clinical lecturers were expected to lead yet were too junior and inexperienced to effect wider change (Macfarlane et al., 2002). Plsek and Wilson (2001) argue that leaders should recognize that change occurs naturally in systems and that individuals engage or resist for a variety of reasons but resistance should not be seen as synonymous with rejection (see Chapter 9).

Needs for control

Even continuous change can disrupt the normal course of events and the smooth running of systems. Davis (1997: iii) claims that images of change frequently evoke feelings across a wide range of emotions, most notably a fear that changes will precipitate chaos and loss of control. Losing control and autonomy over work content and context creates resistance as those involved desperately attempt to make sense of changes. Support mechanisms in terms of participation, provision of information and skills are vital to enable people to regain their feelings of safety (Nadler, 1993) and leader activity should be concerned with helping individuals to interpret emerging change (Rhydderch et al., 2004). Jarrett (2003) also notes that transformational change is often outside organizational control. Change may make some systems irrelevant, inappropriate or even redundant. It is often difficult to monitor performance during rapid change when roles and responsibilities are fractured and, in the common experience of 'top-down' change in healthcare, Rhydderch et al. (2004) suggest that ownership needs to be promoted at the individual and team level to reduce tensions and redress power imbalances.

Process approach

Building further on the emergent approach to change, there are strong arguments that only a continuous and reflective process will be able to improve and sustain change and has the capacity to enable choice in content and methods to build the consensus that is so vital for success (Plsek and Wilson, 2001). Balfour and Clarke (2001) also suggest that whatever strategy is used, the change process should be cyclical so it can be continually refined in the light of reflection, evaluation and review and can deal with 'emergent processes' (Coghlan, 2007: 339) and unexpected and unpredictable outcomes (Burnes, 1996).

In Lewin's action research model (see Figure 2.1), there is deliberate overlapping of action and reflection which is designed to allow changes in plans as people learn from their experiences. Change practitioners and the group involved continue moving through this cycle until they have exhausted the options and found a solution to the problem that they initially identified (Dickens and Watkins, 1999). This replicates Kolb's (1984) learning cycle – ideas about problems are formulated, these are then tested and the effects are evaluated 'since learning is in effect, little more than the management of change' (Pryjmachuk, 1996: 204). Involvement is also implied since people have a greater tendency to support what they have helped to create (Hedley et al., 2003) even if true learning is seen as disruptive (Hendry, 1996). This cycle takes advantage of the naturally occurring creativity embedded (but rarely tapped) in groups and organizations (Plsek and Wilson, 2001). McWilliam and Ward-Griffin (2006) note that even ongoing team meetings enable those involved in change an opportunity for 'reflection-on-action' to uncover values, processes and factors considered relevant for progress.

This cyclical process can be seen in Weick and Quinn's view of how continuous change emerges:

> Repeated acts of improvisation involving simultaneous composition and execution, repeated acts of translation that convert ideas into artifacts that fit purposes at hand, or repeated acts of learning that enlarge, strengthen, or shrink the repertoire of responses. (Weick and Quinn, 1999: 377)

This involves a number of important processes including: 'Change through ongoing variations in practice, cumulation of variations, continuity in place of dramatic discontinuity, continuous disequilibrium as variations beget variations, and no beginning or end point' (Weick and Quinn, 1999: 377).

The process is evident in McWilliam and Ward-Griffin's study (2006) which reports that participants constantly interpret and reinterpret the proposed changes in terms with which they are familiar, slowly constructing and reconstructing their everyday life experience. The key organizational activities which enable these elements to operate successfully are information gathering, communication and learning (Bamford and Forrester, 2003), implicit in the process approach in Figure 6.4 and derived from the management model in Figure 4.1. Jarrett (2003: 28) notes that to create shared direction 'communication, communication, communication' should be used. Perfection is never achieved; rather, this approach should be seen as an ongoing 'process of perfecting' (Orgland, 1997: 26).

Action research and change

In action research, change is not done to people but by them (Massey and Williams, 2006) and the emphasis on social interactions and interpersonal processes implies that a high degree of trust and openness is necessary between researchers and participants (Hartley et al., 1997). Weick and Quinn (1999: 370) quoting Dunphy (1996) observe

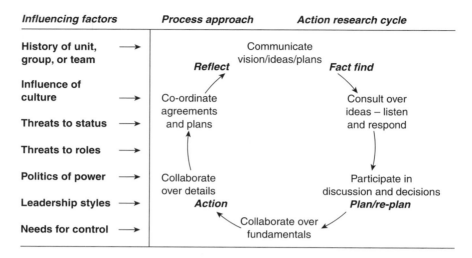

Figure 6.5   Dynamic model of managing change and action research

Source: derived from Parkin (1999a) with permission of the *British Journal of Community Nursing.*

'that the ideal model of an effectively functioning socio-technical system is "a representative democratic community composed of semi-autonomous work groups with the ability to learn continuously through participative action research"'. Hartley et al. (1997) and Hendry (1996) also note that action research is particularly suited to the development of organizational processes where continuous improvement is desired but where outcomes may be complex and unexpected. Action research also recognizes that process goals are as important as research outcomes (Seymour and Davies, 2002) (see Box 6.1).

In responding to Burnes' contention that an emergent model is inappropriate in a bureaucratic 'role' culture, this may be true at the 'macro' level, but at the 'meso' or 'micro' level (see Table 6.2) such as ward, unit or service level, the action research studies cited in this text imply that change can be achieved within large bureaucracies as a result of participative procedures and interactions at local level (Rhydderch et al., 2004), (see Figure 6.5 and Box 6.2)

Box 6.2

Overview

Knightbridge et al. (2006) report on the first phase of a larger project to examine the provision of care for people with complex mental health needs across an extensive group of stakeholders in an Australian community. There is a background of fragmentation of service providers, lack of capacity and unproductive attitudes maintaining the status quo. This study reports the community needs assessment process.

Aims

1 Develop a shared understanding of how this group is cared for.
2 Identify obstacles to better service provision.
3 Identify ways of overcoming obstacles.
4 Identify processes to evaluate programmes from (3).

First exploratory phase

Seventy-one representatives from 53 care provider organizations took part in seven 90-minute focus groups. Groups were audio-taped and data transcribed. Representatives covered care workers, managers, consumers and carers. The data generated focused on defining complex needs, barriers to effective delivery and designing improvements.

Decision and action

Data on definitions (74 items) were condensed into representative statements by independent raters and reproduced into a Likert-type survey ready for the second phase. The solutions (108 items) were transferred onto numbered cards (1–108) for priority sorting.

Second exploratory phase

Focus groups met again and completed the Likert survey and engaged in concept mapping through sorting the solutions into clusters of related themes.

Findings

Four main themes were produced:

1 Reduce fragmentation – less complicated cases were preferred by providers to meet performance indicators. Complex cases were more important but were avoided to enhance productivity. Work was focused on rational, economic and political bases. Providers adhered to strict role definitions.
2 Enhance integrative management – the principles of case management should be applied to promote continuity.
3 Community attitudes – perjorative attitudes regarding certain types of problems, judgements about certain coping strategies and professional blind-spots and rivalries contributed to access difficulties and victim blaming attitudes.
4 Lack of resources – systems of miscommunication caused poor information exchange and a mismatch between what was envisioned and what was implemented.

Summary

- Fragmentation is inherent in complex systems.
- Organizing services around conventional specialisms prevents a holistic approach.
- Structures need to promote inter-agency co-operation and use holistic models of care.

(Continued)

(Continued)

- Providers should work collaboratively with consumers in assessments.
- The case management model is seen as beneficial for inter-agency co-operation.
- Provision of multi-agency training is important.

Future phases

Develop the explanatory model through continuing the participative process, create local advisory groups to monitor progress, and continue regular consultative forums to engage wider providers. These parameters will continually emerge as the project progresses.

Conclusion

Ultimately, successful change can and does occur through both planned and emergent approaches and there are no universal rules to follow and no 'one best way' as Burnes (1996: 11) puts it. However, in healthcare, there is continuous pressure to increase knowledge and skills, to improve performance and to demonstrate greater transparency, accountability and involvement of patients and clients. In this environment a 'stop-start' approach would be inappropriate and restrictive. Organizations and professional staff groups move at varying paces. Large bureaucratic organizations are slower to respond and should not hold back those entities and groups who embrace change willingly.

Chapter summary

- Implementing change can be messy, difficult and the effects short-lived.
- Episodic 'planned' change is generally 'top-down' and used in larger organizations.
- Continuous change is seen as a cyclical 'bottom-up' process.
- Powerful influencing factors affect the uptake and success of change initiatives.
- A positive view sees change as a learning opportunity.

7

Organizational and Professional Cultures in Healthcare

Introduction

If management and leadership are the obvious, visible and concrete features of the change implementation process then organizational and professional cultures are the more covert side of the coin. Yet even suggesting management and leadership as being separate from organizational culture is itself problematic since the actions of leaders and managers are likely, albeit unwittingly, to be influenced and even controlled by the predominant culture in which they work.

In healthcare, where there are numerous occupational and professional groups (Brooks and Brown, 2002), the cultural demarcations between them, which are magnified both in distinctiveness and significance, are likely to have an even greater effect in controlling behaviours, performance and reactions to change. There are therefore robust arguments that practitioners who plan to implement change must pay close attention to understanding the strength and character of their prevailing organizational and professional culture to determine what actions, initiatives and outcomes are desirable and possible. Whether this extends to 'managing' organizational culture is contentious and highly debateable. Indeed, many of the 'planned' reforms in the NHS over the first decade of the twenty-first century have argued that, in addition to structural factors, focusing on and 'managing' organizational culture is the major key to achieving successful reform. However, in many of the guiding policy documents the notions of 'structure' and 'culture', though inextricably entwined, are frequently used synonymously, interchangeably and without explanation. For example *Shifting the Balance of Power within the NHS: Securing Delivery* states:

> Changing the culture and structure of the NHS ... is needed to support and empower patients, the public and frontline staff. We need to change the way we work at all levels. Structural changes to devolve power and responsibility to frontline organizations ... and

changes to the culture and working practices within organizations to devolve decisions to frontline staff [are required]. (DH, 2001a: 12)

Similarly, from *Shifting the Balance of Power: The Next Steps*:

Achieving our vision for the NHS will involve all these elements of cultural and organizational change with the key elements being …:

- Changing the NHS culture and structure by devolving power and decision-making to frontline staff and Primary Care Trusts led by clinicians and local people. (DH, 2002d: 4)

In conflating culture and structure in this way, there is an implication that they are similar entities which are objective – even physical – and can be observed, examined, managed and 'improved'. Thus when staff engage in 'new ways of working' (to improve the quality of patient care for example), managers (and politicians) can claim this as evidence that the 'change in culture' (DH, 2001a: 23) has been achieved and the policy vindicated.

Further policies point to a variety of cultural configurations including an 'involving' and a 'supportive' culture (DH, 2002e: 17, 40), a 'culture of blame' and a 'communication culture between doctors and patients' (Healthcare Commission, 2006: 34, 73), the last requiring 'improvement' through adopting a more 'open' system.

The NHS Improvement Plan (DH, 2004a) identifies cultures of 'waiting' (2004a: 11), 'reporting' (2004a: 21), 'patient safety' (2004a: 31) and a 'culture responsive to change' (2004a: 63). This last culture is to be achieved through making structural changes in 'improving team-working, appraisal and diversity'.

Creating a Patient-led NHS states:

Becoming a truly patient-led NHS will require more than just changes in systems. There need to be changes in how the system works and how people behave and a change in culture where everything is measured by its impact on patients. (DH, 2005: 24)

The term 'culture' in these examples appears to be devoid of any clarity of meaning and used as accusative shorthand for inefficiencies and criticisms of staff behaviours. This transfers the focus of 'change' onto staff and their actions rather than any constraints imposed by the structure and systems of the service. Grey (2005) argues that embracing the concept of 'organizational culture', derived from American business theory, is designed to create shifts away from a public sector ethos to a more business-like orientation. The underlying message is that if the 'culture' is changed then the behaviours and attitudes of staff to, for example, patient safety, waiting, or communication, will improve; a point made forcibly in the *NHS Plan*:

Old-fashioned demarcations between staff, restricted opening and operating times, outdated systems, unnecessarily complex procedures and a lack of training all combine to create a culture where the convenience of the patient can come a poor second to the convenience of the system. (DH, 2000a: 15)

Many contemporary writers would disagree with this conflation and view the suggestion that an organization's culture can be re-engineered, manipulated and mandated by managerial actions and diktats to suit corporate plans as overly simplistic and modernist (Davies et al., 2000; Scott et al., 2003), outdated (Worthington, 2004) and wrong-headed (Grey, 2005). Degeling and Carr (2004: 403) argue that many current policies assume that healthcare leaders can act independently of the organizational culture which is seen primarily as the outcome of senior managers' policies, plans and actions 'as though it is simply a vehicle for senior management to "colonise" the minds of staff'. A view asserted in '*A First Class Service*' (DH, 1998: 72) which states 'we want to create a culture in the NHS which celebrates and encourages success and innovation'. Degeling and Carr (2004: 404) claim this view disregards the contribution and actions of other staff members and the cumulative 'historical residue of events' which is so powerful in controlling behaviour and ways of thinking. Even though there is agreement that to achieve lasting change in healthcare a change in culture is required, it is counterproductive to attempt it by attacking the existing culture (Carroll and Quijada, 2004). It is therefore timely that, having considered management and leadership in implementing change, this discussion moves to examine the 'cloudy domain of organizational culture' (Buchanan and Badham, 1999: 55).

Chapter 4 proposed that management was concerned with the process of balancing and co-ordinating the knowledge, interests and needs of employees to enable the group or organization to meet its goals. This chapter argues that achieving the interests and needs of groups and organizations can be enhanced or constrained by the strength and power of their culture. It will therefore consider:

- through an 'idealized' account, how organizational and professional cultures develop;
- the meaning of the term 'culture' in relation to groups and organizations;
- the effects of culture on the change process;
- the role and significance of professional cultures in healthcare.

How organizational culture develops

Level 1 – the new, single group

Several people sitting together in a doctor's waiting room or in a train carriage may experience limited and generalized interaction but collectively they do not constitute a 'group' since there is no task to achieve and no need to develop social relations or 'patterns of behaviour'.

Schein (2004) suggests that within hours of an unstructured group of individuals coming together to achieve a goal (for example army recruits or medical students) there emerges spontaneous interaction which gradually leads to patterns and norms of behaviour which eventually grow into and form the 'culture' of that group. The patterns and norms emerge from both verbal and non-verbal interactions between members which, over time, become tacitly shared and understood by the group as signifying its identity and coherence.

Blau and Scott (1963: 7) discuss the example of a 'group of boys who hang around the drugstore'. If the group is small enough for each member to be in direct contact with one another, it will develop its status hierarchies; flows of influence; degrees of co-operation, respect, hostility and attraction; its leaders and followers; its central and peripheral characters. Over time these elements combine to become its culture, its 'informal' relations. This 'social enclave' (Chan, 1997: 94) may be described by outsiders as a 'team', 'club', 'gang', 'pack', 'clan', 'tribe', 'brotherhood', 'fellowship', 'regiment' – terms which themselves are imbued with social, gender, and class connotations carrying predetermined interpretive 'cultural' significance. As more are drawn to the group, opinions and assumptions will pluralize, threatening cohesion and creating more difference, fragmentation and potential conflict; the culture will change, diversify and weaken. Alternatively, if members wish to retain exclusivity and cohesion and prevent dilution, such as in a 'clan' or 'corporate' culture (Chan, 1997) then high social barriers to entry are set through initiations, skills, standards and qualifications; strong, clear values, beliefs and boundaries are drawn through rites of passage; covert language, dress and behaviour codes develop to aid identification; to maintain member loyalty, strong, contractual bonds and sanctions against rule-breaking are devised.

Thus Bauman explains the role of culture in his description of 'in' and 'out' groups:

> An out-group is precisely that imaginary opposition to itself which the in-group needs for its self-identity, for its cohesiveness, for its inner solidarity and emotional security … for the sake of coherence and integration of the group it must postulate an enemy to draw and guard its own boundaries and to secure loyalty and co-operation within. (Bauman, 1990: 41–2)

The longer and more intensively the group interacts, the more complex its tasks and problems, the more conflict, threats and crises that have to be managed and the more vital its memberships' needs, so its 'way of life' will emerge, develop and crystallize, maturing and strengthening to produce a powerful sense of belonging and identity.

Level 2 – multiplying groups, developing orgnizations

Blau and Scott (1963: 7) continue that if the group of boys has no specific objectives requiring co-ordination, tasks are relatively straightforward, procedures simple and membership is clear, then there is little need for any structure or 'formal' organization. If however they wish to transform themselves into a football club then they need to develop 'administrative machinery', become more explicitly 'organized' with structures, processes, procedures and divisions of labour (chair, secretary, treasurer, committee members).

Extending Blau and Scott's example: to graduate from kicking a ball in the park to playing as members of a league, the 'group' must transform into a 'club' and 'team'; it must develop team roles, positions and skills, learn to 'play by the rules' – this includes its own informal internal rules, the formally agreed game's rules and the 'official' football league's regulations. The league's controlling regulations develop through wider social influences, protracted discussions and negotiations by senior and respected members (leaders) and representatives of the teams. Regulations become the means for controlling behaviour (a code of conduct) in co-ordination and competition with others. In this way the 'league' and the way it works becomes a representation of both the 'teams' and the 'game' which itself reflects the beliefs and values of the individuals who were once 'hanging around the drugstore'. Break the regulations and the team will be disciplined, demoted, struck off or 'lose its licence to practice'. If teams played by their own rules, anarchy would result; the league would lose its authority; its organization would disintegrate and it would be unable to achieve its purpose. As more teams and countries apply to join the league and it spreads internationally, it becomes 'complex by design' (Blau and Scott, 1963: 7). As Pettigrew (1979: 574) argues, new organizations (or groups or teams) represent 'transition processes from no beliefs to new beliefs, from no rules to new rules, from no culture to new culture'.

Furthermore these behavioural guidelines, the 'rules of the game', are not biologically or genetically transmitted but are a 'learned group phenomenon' (Hendry, 1996: 624). This implies that culture is organic, a dynamic and adaptive rather than a static phenomenon and is amenable to change depending on the power, variety and mix of individuals and groups. It spreads through symbolic interaction, not randomly but spontaneously and unpredictably between and within individuals and groups and throughout an organization. Where formal guidelines (regulations) are insufficient or unsatisfactory, informal practices will develop which may influence the 'formal' structural arrangements. Since it is 'socially created, socially maintained and socially transformed' (Manley, 2000: 38), culture is unmanageable and uncontrollable (Wallace et al., 1999; Grey, 2005) and 'unbounded' (Savage, 2000: 231).

Level 3 – maturing groups, complex organizations

The group of boys may play in the park in jeans and T-shirts but when playing in a league this would be insufficient, irregular and 'unprofessional'. It needs a team name and a uniform or 'strip' to delineate its identity and to distinguish it from others – this involves choosing a logo, a colour scheme and sponsorship. Decisions over a colour scheme may reflect religious and national identity such as 'All Blacks'; decisions over a name and logo may signify qualities indicating strength or competitiveness such as 'British Lions' or 'Springboks' and become 'symbolic' of the team. These decisions may evolve through discussions, negotiations and arguments. Hence words and the meaning of words become the main creators of cultural symbols. The strip and logo become the visible symbols – the short-hand or icon – of the group's value system and self identity; they serve to distinguish it from all others; they create its difference and its reality. Schein (2004) uses the term 'artifacts' and argues that these outward signs of behaviours, products, style and creations should not be seen as the culture of the group but are the visible expressions of deeper values and beliefs; they are easy to observe but it is difficult to decipher their rationale and the cultural beliefs underlying their creation.

As time passes into history, the original members move on and, as the organization matures, the rationale for choices becomes forgotten; new members and followers then see the symbols as 'traditions' and feel that it has always been like this – to change would be a denial of history, identity and heritage. As the symbols embed and become the group's core identity, they become unchallengeable, immovable and barriers to change and progress.

A group's social history also develops rituals and ceremonies. These have particularly significant meanings and serve to constrain and adhere the membership.

Extending the metaphor, the All Blacks rugby team begin each match with the 'Haka', a powerful, symbolic ceremonial exhibition designed to instil strength, determination, solidarity and cohesion in adversity in the team and intimidate the opposition:

> More than any aspect of Maori culture, this complex dance is an expression of the passion, vigour and identity of the race. Haka is not merely a past-time of the Maori but was also a custom of high social importance in the welcoming and entertainment of visitors. Tribal reputations rose and fell on their ability to perform the haka.
>
> Haka reflected the concerns and issues of the time, of defiance and protest, of factual occurrences and events at any given time.
>
> The centrality of the haka within All Black rugby tradition is not a recent development … its mystique has evolved along with the fierce determination, commitment and high level skill which has been the hallmark of New Zealand's national game. (NZRU, 2003)

The Haka tells a mythical story of survival and triumph of the Maori tribe and is exclusively identified with the All Blacks as the expression of their culture – their underlying character and ideology. Such can be the identification of culture with an organization (or sport with a nation) that Pacanowsky and O'Donnell-Trujillo (1982: 126) argue that 'culture is not something an organisation has, culture is something an organisation is'; it 'defines the group' (Schein, 2004: 14); it 'sets it apart' (Bauman, 1990: 148).

Hence Brown (1998) suggests that organizational culture originates from the:

* prevailing societal and national culture;
* background, status, class and gender orientations of members;
* vision, management style and personality of the founder/leader (for example in dimensions of autocracy and democracy or freedom and control);
* needs and aspirations of its members;
* type of 'business' and nature of the 'business environment' (for example the level of stability, uncertainty or competition).

What is organizational culture?

Attempts to define culture can be traced through anthropological studies of human populations over many centuries (Helman, 1990) and yet its nature remains highly elusive and contested (Hyde and Davies, 2004); it is difficult to study (Scott et al., 2003), genuinely complex and difficult to understand (Schein, 1985) and no consensus exists as to the range and definition of its variables (Davies et al., 2000). David Glencross, Chairman of the Independent Television Commission once claimed that when the government heard the word 'culture' its likely response was to reach for a dictionary (Glencross, 1988), yet

Helman cites a definition from as early as 1871 (Tylor cited in Helman, 1990). Hofstede (1998: 478) lists 51 constructs which are used in the literature to describe people's 'collective programming of the mind'. Wallace et al. (1999) claim that Blau and Scott (1963) were amongst the first to describe organizations as being both 'formal' and 'informal' and that the first major analysis of the 'informal' dimension was by Peters in 1978 marking the start of the 'appropriation of culture by management theorists' (Savage, 2000: 232).

A year later Pettigrew asserts that the purpose of his paper is to highlight the 'expressive aspects of organizational life ... which have not yet been integrated into the theoretical language of organizational behaviour' (1979: 579–80), yet Grey (2005: 67) claims that culture became '*the* word' within organizations throughout the 1980s and 1990s indicating that culture as applied to organizations has had a short but intensive analytical history.

The term is derived from the French *culture* and Latin *cultura* meaning 'growing' or 'cultivation' and therefore has a developmental and evolutionary property. Whereas an individual would possess a 'character' or 'personality', the term 'culture' is reserved for groups of people acknowledging the influence of the common, shared and mutually understood dimensions emerging from human interaction. Schein (1985) claims that culture, as a learned product of group experience, can only be found where there is a definable group with a significant history. Culture is therefore a social (and socially constructed) rather than an individual phenomenon (Hofstede, 1998; Manley, 2000).

Schein (2004: 70–1) and Brown (1998) assert that the major foci of individuals' interactions within groups are concerned with:

- making a situation personally safe and rewarding;
- managing personal issues around:
  - inclusion and identity;
  - authority, control, power and influence;
  - acceptance and intimacy.

As discussed above, groups are usually formed for a purpose and Schein argues that in order to achieve 'personal safety' and 'feelings of inclusion' it is necessary for individuals to find out what the group's task and purpose is, and its suitability and appropriateness, hence they will look for:

- indications that they will 'fit in';
- reassurance that they are doing the right things;
- approval that they are behaving in a way which is acceptable to others.

This guidance may come from the leaders or 'authority figures' (the originator or co-ordinator of the group) or a designated 'mentor' or teacher with the aim of developing a 'psychological bond' and a sense of 'belonging' (Avery, 2004: 119). In this way the leader has the opportunity to form, create and design the emerging culture, to 'build from the top down' (Pettigrew, 1979: 574). This has led Schein (1985: 317) to claim that culture can not only be created, embedded and strengthened by leaders but that the leadership role can be simplified to '*the manipulation of culture*'.

From an anthropological perspective, Helman defines culture as:

> A set of guidelines (both explicit and implicit) which individuals inherit as members of a particular society, and which tells them how to *view* the world, how to experience it *emotionally*, and how to *behave* in it in relation to other people … It also provides them with a way of transmitting these guidelines to the next generation – by the use of symbols, language, art and ritual … Culture can be seen as an inherited 'lens', through which individuals perceive and understand the world that they inhabit, and learn how to live within it. (Helman, 1990: 2)

Defining 'organizational' culture, Hofstede (1998: 478) calls it 'the collective programming of the mind which distinguishes the members of one organization from another'.

Although the concepts below are not exhaustive, writers (Blau and Scott, 1963; Pettigrew, 1979; Hofstede, 1998; Morgan, 1998; Martins and Terblanche, 2003; Schein, 2004; Mannion et al., 2005) agree that the basic concepts of organizational culture are concerned with:

Beliefs Knowledge and assumptions (thoughts) about the world (people and objects) and how it works; these vary in importance, endurance and certainty.

Values Strong, underlying and inexplicit predispositions (feelings) about judging and preferring certain states of affairs over others, for example regarding right and wrong or acceptable and unacceptable behaviour, conduct and ethical codes; they are the 'ends' of human conduct which justify behaviour. Values provide internal consistency across thoughts and emotions and are implied through conduct.

Identity Shared understanding about the nature of the organization, what it is and what it stands for. Actions become supportive rather than competitive when faced with extreme threats to identity (Chan, 1997).

Image Identity as understood by those outside the organization – for example whether it is efficient, ethical or a 'good' employer.

Norms Shared expectations of behaviour and rules of conduct such as presentation, dress codes, time-keeping and attending meetings. These denote what is desirable and appropriate in certain situations and act as unstated guidance, social regulation and mechanisms of control; they are the 'means' of achieving the value 'ends'.

Ideology The dominant set of interrelated assumptions about the social world, which are unconsciously organized into an internally consistent hierarchy and which explain, motivate and justify why the major shared understandings 'make sense' to those in the organization. It can determine consistent and persistent responses to solving problems, decision-making and social arrangements. Ideology is highly resistant to change.

These concepts emphasize the central role that 'agreement' has on moral values for maintaining social order which gives a group its solidarity, its 'collective conscience', its 'collectively accepted meanings' and 'sense of orientation' (Pettigrew, 1979: 574), its 'unique cultural blueprint' (Paton and McCalman, 2000: 41). Furthermore, since they are considered valid they are taught to new members as the 'correct way to perceive, think, and feel in relation to those problems' (Schein, 1985: 9). In this way organizations and groups perpetuate their culture through the individuals they attract, the leaders they choose and the behaviours they value, promote and punish. From these concepts, Pettigrew cites 'symbol, language, ritual and myth' as the 'offspring' of culture and of these, he claims that 'symbols' are the most significant frame of reference as they include language, rituals and ideologies and identify individuals as '*creators* and *managers of meaning*' (1979: 572).

The effects of culture on the change process

Buchanan and Badham (1999) conclude that taken together these concepts establish a fabric of norms and expectations that not only shape attitudes and behaviour but also influence the distribution of power and privilege across the organization's membership. They are a powerful guide to workers' decision-making processes and action and can be the 'antecedents of performance' (Hyde and Davies, 2004: 1408). Hendry (1996: 622) and Grey (2005) go further and suggest that the functional consequences of culture are evident in exerting conformity, exercising control, constraining and prescribing behaviour (what can be said, done and thought) and deterring learning, and, that because the culture becomes embedded in ordinary processes of work and interaction, these have a tendency toward inertia, reduction of variance and promotion of work routinization. As Schein (1985: 314) claims 'Culture controls the manager more than the manager controls culture ... it influences *everything* the manager does'. In this way culture can militate against change and impinge on individualism and autonomy. Workers' performance is a result of the structural arrangements and service design which themselves are a result of the assumptions and ideology of the organization. Routinization of work can become a means to create order, personal security and reduce anxiety (socalled 'comfort zones') but this can lead to repetition and the development of ritual which itself becomes symbolic (Helman, 1990). Pettigrew states that a ritual is the symbolic use of bodily movements to communicate a specific message.

To take an example, Bone (2003) illustrates the strength of diplomatic culture within the United Nations (UN). In the shuttle diplomacy at the start of the Iraq war in 2003, Mr Blair, the British Prime Minister, requested that the UN Secretary-General meet him at Kennedy Airport to discuss the forthcoming UN vote. Bone reports that the request provoked horror at UN Headquarters and explained that protocol (the embodiment of cultural values) is so specific that it even prescribes whether the Secretary-General greets dignitaries in his office or meets them at the lift. He will meet heads of state at the lift but those of lesser rank such as foreign ministers must walk the corridor. The ritual of 'walking the corridor' *symbolizes* the hierarchical status and power structures that need to be preserved in this cultural context and which must be decoded by participants – it is not the action (of walking the corridor) which is important but what that action conveys. The ritual communicates the message, making difficult verbal explanations redundant. For the UN chief to walk the corridor for a foreign minister (or leave the building to meet a head of state) would set a dangerous precedent. He did not go to Kennedy Airport for fear it would make him appear as 'Mr Blair's poodle'. As Pettigrew (1979: 576) argues: 'What ritual [as a symbol of culture] can say is that ... these are the central or peripheral values, the dominant or marginal people, the highly prized or less important goals'.

Culture or structure?

It is argued above that recent NHS policies appear to use culture and structure interchangeably and synonymously but, though they are interdependent and they cannot
exist separately (Procter et al., 1999) there are important distinctions. Indeed they can
be separated only artificially for the purpose of analysis.

Paton and McCalman (2000: 42) discuss a 'cultural web' of tangible (structural) and
intangible (cultural) aspects (Blau and Scott (1963) use the terms 'formal' and 'informal'
respectively) – the tangible being the physical manifestations of the hidden 'intangibles'.

In young organizations (or football teams) the visible, tangible aspects which include
administrative systems, roles and routines, quality control, reward mechanisms, organizational boundaries, communication systems and even the fabric and design of its
buildings and services (or the colour and logo of a strip) are not the organization's culture. These develop contemporaneously and interactively with its culture as its physical
embodiment, the manifestation of the hidden, deeper cultural assumptions – they 'represent' the culture and therefore can have profound symbolic meaning (Schein, 2004).
Viewed in this way, structural aspects are often designed in the wake of cultural values.
As Blau and Scott argue (1963: 6) 'unofficial practices (culture) furnish guides for decisions long before the formal rules (structure) have been adapted to the changing
circumstances'.

As organizations and their structures develop, so they influence, limit and control the
development and dynamics of cultural practices which themselves are shaped by new
people and new structures, which are shaped by social practices in an iterative cycle.
Schein (2004: 262) claims that as organizations mature their structures become the 'primary culture-creating mechanisms' that constrain and control employees' behaviour.
Therefore attempting to change or manage culture within a 'top-down' project focusing
on visions and missions as suggested in the NHS policies noted above may have no or
only limited effect on actions and behaviours. Likewise, attempts at changing cultural
beliefs will not necessarily have material effects on organizational structures in mature
organizations (see Chapter 11); a point articulated by an NHS Locality Manager in a
trust aiming to 'create' a culture of middle management empowerment:

> The minute you do anything wrong … they [Personnel] will slap your wrists. And you say
> 'Hang on a minute. On the one hand you empower us and the next you police us'. They police
> us now, and so you end up with a subculture that says, 'Don't tell them'. So we don't tell them
> anymore and do our own thing. Then they find out and say, 'You can't do that'. And we say,
> 'Well, we got fed up of asking for permission, so we're doing it now'. (Procter et al., 1999: 253)

Here, the mature, bureaucratic, organizational structure becomes an impediment to
enabling the culture change desired by the organization and the actors become subversive to achieve their ends. The change initiative therefore failed as the Locality Managers
were 'empowered' only as far as they followed the centrally laid down organizational
regulations (Procter et al., 1999). Similarly, discussing a 'cultural change' programme in
a European university, Diefenbach (2007: 132) showed that staff did not openly resist

imposed change but coped with it in a tactical way; they 'listen to all the change rhetoric, make up their minds – and find ways to bypass it in their daily routines'.

From the above discussion, several points can be made regarding the term 'culture':

1   It is informal, invisible, intrinsic and implicit and therefore can only be *deduced* from observing a range of artefacts, symbols and behaviours.
2   It develops through social interaction, informal networks and meanings created by workers rather than through 'culture change programmes', away days or mission statements.
3   It is maintained and perpetuated through:
    (a)   selection processes (including self, peer and qualification criteria);
    (b)   formal and informal socialization and enculturation processes (including mentoring, and educational and training courses);
    (c)   reinforcment of values through professional body registration, licensing, regulatory frameworks and codes of conduct.
4   Where people share a strong set of common goals and vision about their enterprise, such as in 'clan' or 'corporate' cultures (Chan, 1997), they are more likely to show commitment and work co-operatively to achieve ends without the need for external management controls. Leaders and politicians therefore believe that if they can 'manage' organizational culture they can control the way staff work (Grey, 2005).
5   Where there is a wide range of professional and occupational groups (such as in healthcare) universal recognition and adherence to cultural values is dissipated and weakened.
6   The task of leaders, therefore, is to make decisions and create conditions, systems and structures that reflect those cultures which motivate and enable workers to achieve their aims (Morgan, 1998).

Professional culture in healthcare

The aim of this section is to apply the above discussion, through the use of examples, to the role of occupational and professional cultures in healthcare and assess their influence on managing change.

There is a high level of consensus over the main objectives of UK healthcare provision (DH, 2000a: Darzi, 2007). Davies et al. (2000) and Merali (2003) agree that there are not only long-standing cultural values, including a belief in a universal, comprehensive and free (at point of delivery) service and a commitment to improve health outcomes, but also newer developing values such as a belief in equity, centrality of patient care, use of evidence, and acceptance of quality controls and audit procedures. Furthermore, Preston et al. (1996: 347) argue that the culture of health services in the UK is influenced by national culture, historical traditions, public perceptions and media reporting, professional perceptions (of doctors, nurses, midwives and managers) and individual perceptions, which together create a socially constructed 'symbolic-meaningful system'. Yet Worthington (2004) argues that the NHS is a highly dispersed and fragmented organization and the one element that binds its employees is their respective occupational affiliations and that these act as more powerful control mechanisms than the wider organizational values.

Carroll and Quijada (2004: ii17) agree that professional cultures within healthcare are distinctive and that a hospital cannot be seen as a single culture, rather it is a 'fragmented collection of occupational cultures'. Drife and Johnson (1995: 1054) also describe the NHS as 'a multi-cultural society', with each profession, occupational and specialty group having its own unique identity, subculture, characteristics and aims. They claim that the potential for conflict arising from these differences is almost limitless.

An editorial from *The Times* discussing the implementation of the *NHS Plan* agrees:

> There is no doubt that the various professional bodies within the health service guard their autonomy and the distinctive roles that each has played inside the NHS, with unusual vigour. Doctors and consultants often tend to dismiss innovations, such as NHS Direct, and to view with scepticism the notion that nurses could take over tasks traditionally performed by doctors. (*The Times*, 2000)

Brookes and Brown (2002: 344) term this 'tribalism' which they claim is ingrained in healthcare, creating rich breeding grounds for ceremonial activity, the investment of considerable emotional capital and a great deal of routinized behaviour aimed at preserving demarcation lines, roles and territories. The Bristol Hospital Inquiry Report (Kennedy, 2001: 266) found that the cultures of doctors, nurses and managers 'are so distinct and internally closely-knit that the words, "tribe" and "tribal" were commonly used' to describe them.

These comments reflect enduring problems of symbolic relevance in healthcare: the hierarchical role structure and status, the hard-won and fiercely protected knowledge, skills and expertise which prescribe how different professional groups work, act, and what they have responsibility for and the perceptions of their relative importance to the overall goals of the healthcare system (Preston et al., 1996). Kennedy summarizes:

> This old-style paternalism is evident in the adherence to the idea of hierarchy ... the continued existence of a hierarchical approach within and between the healthcare professions is a significant cultural weakness ... these aspects of the current culture of the NHS are simply inappropriate. They are a product of dated professional self-images. (Kennedy, 2001: 268–9)

There is evidence (Mannion et al., 2005) of changes to many of these aspects which indicates that culture can and does change but only in certain circumstances such as through a major shift in how a profession views itself (Ferlie and Shortell, 2001). A more detailed examination of change strategies is discussed in Chapter 11.

Managerial culture

Significant aspects of managerial orientations were discussed in Chapter 4.

Merali (2003) studied 28 managers from NHS Trusts in London and found that they believe that all NHS workers shared their 'altruistic' core values but that the public did not see them as altruistic, which they think unfair. He reports that managers are convinced that the public believe doctors and nurses were the only professionals who were motivated to provide care to society. In endorsing Bauman's (1990) notion of 'in' and 'out' groups, managers also believe that clinicians, politicians and the media actively propagate a 'poor image' of them – clinicians in an attempt to increase their power, and politicians in a cynical move to identify a scapegoat to take the blame for failures and inadequacies of the healthcare system. This distrust illustrates the enduring 'major cultural divide' between healthcare organizations' clinical and managerial cultures (Ferlie and Shortell, 2001: 293).

Medical and nursing culture

One area of difference between doctors' and nurses' belief systems is in the fundamental identity of being a professional. Walby et al. (1994: 52) found that many nurses saw a professional as being 'someone accountable for their practice, guided by rules and monitored by senior professionals'. Rules were seen as protective and providing security. Within medicine however, a professional was seen as someone who takes responsibility for their own decisions and actions and rules are seen as restrictive. The clash of cultures is evidenced in doctors thinking that nurses do not take responsibility and nurses viewing doctors as getting away with 'slip-shod' practice that would be unacceptable in nursing.

Whereas in the United States, the 'golden age' of medicine may be over through the curtailing and regulating of professional discretion and autonomy (Carroll and Quijada, 2004: ii16), in the UK, clinician autonomy and its dominance within healthcare remains largely unchanged (Davies et al., 2000: 113). The traditional occupational identity of the medical profession is its autonomy from state control, management regulation or lay interference. Worthington terms this 'the most distinctive and highly prized characteristic' (Worthington, 2004: 63). Doctors operate in a professional culture where control mechanisms exist by mutual consent: influence is shared; the source of power is expertise; and the basic assumption that practitioners have the right to make their own decisions is the cornerstone of medical culture (Carroll and Quijada, 2004) – but this does not apply to all occupational groups in healthcare. Walby et al. (1994) emphasize that if the work of doctors and nurses were unrelated then differences would not matter. However since it is so interdependent, differences in their cultural beliefs make conflict inevitable. Kennedy sums up the dangers:

> An appeal to 'clinical freedom' is a claim that in the care of a patient, the doctor's decision is the determining decision and may not be challenged … the doctrine becomes code for 'doctor knows best'. In a modern healthcare system, where professionals must work in teams, such an approach may be counterproductive. (Kennedy, 2001: 269)

The notion of individual autonomy reinforces both a Western (Worthington, 2004) and a 'masculine' belief that it is the mark of the 'true professional' (Davies, 1995: 56) rather than team-based practice (Worthington, 2004). Davies (1995) explains further that doctors can only claim to be autonomous because of the considerable sustaining and supportive work carried out by nurses and other 'bureaucratic systems' mainly carried out by women.

A second example of the development and role of subcultures within healthcare is the symbol of the 'handover report' in nursing (Holland, 1993) and the 'firm' in medicine (Davies, 1995; Preston et al., 1996) where doctors are organized into specialty groups with the consultant as the leader and role model with a hierarchy of various levels below. Preston et al. (1996) and Holland (1993) note that both 'rituals' become a significant means of cultural transfer in influencing the behaviour, style, attitudes and communication patterns (the collective programming of the mind) of junior staff. The action research study in Box 7.1 shows a laudable attempt to 'widen participation' to medical school for under-represented groups. However the summer school for 16 year olds culminated in the 'grand round' where groups worked in presenting a real patient case study, and in emulating the 'firm', the groups not only became highly competitive but were subjected to the subtle enculturation processes and practices of these specialities.

Box 7.1

Overview

Greenhalgh et al. (2006) report on a UK 'widening-access' study encouraging able 16 year olds from non-traditional backgrounds (lower socio-economic groups, under-represented ethnic minorities, those with non-university educated parents and from state schools) to apply to medical school. Failure to apply and sustain medical study is attributed to lack of confidence, support and motivation; unrealistic images of doctors and medical schools; and self-identity of not being a 'university type'.

Aims

Through action research, to devise and run a week's 'summer school' to promote confidence, professional identity, provide medical role models and an 'insider's view' of the breadth of medicine.

Liaison and recruitment phase

A steering group established including representatives from funders, schools, NHS trusts and medical schools.

Forty pupils (from 19 countries of origin with 16 languages) recruited via recommendations, interviews and personal statements which were transcribed and analysed. Findings presented to steering group, medical students, pupils and parents.

Findings

Pupils suffered from lack of self-determination, confidence, information – little knowledge of primary and chronic care, prevention and rehabilitation; under-estimated their strengths and achievements.

Design phase

The programme was developed and refined following feedback and consultation. Main requirements:

- Hands-on work.
- Ninety per cent of programme taught in small groups.
- High staff–pupil ratio.
- Observation of operations.

Medical students trained as 'buddies'; suitable, inspirational medical lecturers prepared to lead real patient-focused sessions; structured lesson plans devised; staff primed to assist with 'grand round'.

Delivery phase

Medical students acted as mentors, guides and trouble-shooters. Real operations viewed in pairs. End of day de-briefing and risk management.
    The final 'grand round' designed to develop 'peer group bonding' was a key event:

- Groups of 10.
- Interviewed real patients; shared out tasks: locating x-rays, electrocardiographs, histology reports; researched drugs with action and side effects.
- Examined evidence base for medical management and confidentiality.
- Collated and presented evidence to peers, teachers, medical students, staff and parents via PowerPoint.

The 'grand round', symbolic of real life hospital-based medical work generated an 'aura of an escalating (and highly competitive) treasure hunt' (Greenhaigh et al., 2006: 764) with each group trying to outperform others.

Evaluation

Extremely positive feedback by pupils, medical staff and medical students; objectives fully met. Pupils were motivated, mature, interested and keen to learn and work. Medical students were important for creating sense of group camaraderie and bonding.
    Staff provided leadership and vision in capturing teachers' and pupils' priorities and tailor-making the course.

Summary

The type of course provided was instrumental in changing attitudes through:

- social modelling – learning 'bedside manners';
- collective sense making – reframing information until it made sense;
- reframing of identity – moving from 'non university' to 'university' type;
- social drama – becoming caught up in a real story (the 'grand' round).

A third example refers to a study of 'incident reporting' in a UK NHS Trust (Waring, 2004). Patient safety is an important area for organizational learning (see Chapter 8) and healthcare providers have established organization-wide incident reporting procedures. Waring studied five clinical departments: Acute Medicine, Anaesthesia, Surgery, Obstetrics and Rehabilitation and their responses illuminate prevailing subcultural beliefs regarding incidents.

- Acute Medicine and Rehabilitation generally supported risk management, however the clinical leads were disinclined to participate as the system was seen as 'nurse-led, dealing with ward issues and the work of non-medical groups' (Waring, 2004: 349). Though a separate, local procedure was devised, it was abandoned after 3 months.
- Anaesthesia was disinclined to participate in the hospital-wide process preferring to devise its own 'specialty based' system which could be returned anonymously to 'keep it in house as opposed to referring it outside our department' (Waring, 2004: 350).
- General Surgery expressed its unfamiliarity with the reporting system, was unclear about its purpose and expressed some hostility to reporting any incidents to hospital management. Though it did not have a local system, neither did it participate in the wider system preferring schemes that were 'collegial' and offered 'professional development'.
- Obstetrics was the specialty most enthusiastic and supportive of incident reporting: staff are used to reporting and using the hospital system; they experience greater litigation pressures, receive extensive professional education, specialized support, proactive leadership and have a designated 'risk-lead'.

Waring (2004: 351) summarizes that the reporting systems reflect 'distrust in the activities of non-medical groups', a preference for 'professional control and collegiality' and 'the exclusion of non-professional groups' in the evaluation of performance. This study appears to endorse Kinnunen's (1990) study of the three main professional subcultures in primary care. The findings, summarized in Table 7.1, indicate the individualized base of medical subculture in the assumption of 'human relationships'.

More worryingly, as an indication for promoting multi-disciplinary teamwork, in terms of the cultural groups' mutability, all displayed the same assumptions: that members were 'mutable' within their own group but they doubted others, further adding credence to Bauman's (1990) notion of 'in' and 'out' groups.

Midwifery culture

Kirkham (1999) reports on an ethnographic study of the English midwifery service. She uncovers a culture seemingly lost to professional ethics and mutual caring; one that cared highly for clients but spiralled into mutual blame, helplessness, conflict, guilt and oppression when dealing with intra-professional issues (see also Deery, 2005, Box 10.2).

Table 7.1   Influence of health professional cultures on change initiatives

Basic Assumptions	Medical subculture	Nursing subculture	Managerial subculture
Relationships to environment:			
Basic identity	Experts and specialists	Helpers and supporters	Public authorities
Relevant environments	Scientific and technical	Socio-cultural	Economic and political
Position vis-à-vis environments	Dominant	Harmonious and symbiotic	Dominant
Nature of reality and truth			
Verification criteria	Scientific tests and authorities	Traditions and moral dogma	Authorities, rational-legal
Essence of human nature			
Mutability	**In own group, members mutable but doubting others**	**Same**	**Same**
Nature of human relationships			
Relations between people	Individuality, competition	Collaterality, group consensus	Collaterality, autocracy
Relations between organizations	Paternalism, collegial	Participation, delegation	Paternalism, consultation

Source: J. Kinnunen (1990): The importance of organisational culture on development activities in a primary health care organisation. Copyright John Wiley & Sons Limited. Adapted and reproduced with permission.

Particularly this translates into lack of a unified voice and an inability to manage change which could only be achieved by stealth.

Conclusion

Many of the concepts raised in this chapter are revisited and developed further in Chapters 8 and 11, however, in terms of the relevance of action research to organizational culture, Coughlan and Coghlan (2002) argue that changing practice through action research requires a scope of pre-understanding of the corporate (cultural) environment, business conditions, operating systems' structure and dynamics much of which, they claim, is tacit. There is also a need to actively engage in and manage the political dimension of the organization (Williamson and Prosser, 2002a) and work towards developing a culture that emphasizes learning and teamwork (Box 7.2).

Box 7.2

Overview

Cullen et al. (2003) provide an overview of the process of inter-professional education between midwifery and medical students following the merger of the academic divisions of child health, midwifery, obstetrics and gynaecology in a UK university. The merger was designed to create an organizational structure to enhance opportunities for inter-professional collaboration.

Exploratory and planning phase

Multi-professional education is important in cultivating role understanding and facilitating collaborative practice but, if held too early, creates feelings of antagonism and professional rivalry.

A collaborative group of academic midwives and obstetricians was formed and, using 'insider' action research, worked with colleagues and students to identify opportunities to improve and integrate professional roles.

Outcome of phase 1

A strategy was formed to:

- develop team approaches to manage obstetric problems
- develop awareness of each other's roles and knowledge base
- determine future opportunities for integration of midwifery and medical learning.

Action

Developed one session in medical students' 4th year and midwives' final year when students felt more confident of their roles. Midwives participated on three occasions.

Phase 2

Decisions on learning and teaching strategies:

- Students learn best about roles working in small groups.
- Objective Structured Clinical Examination (OSCE) considered the most useful learning approach. OSCE is a series of time-based, interactive stations, each with a facilitator, posing problems which students are asked to solve while being assessed against set criteria.

Action

Teams of 6–8 students were optimum. Hence 90 students participated making the exercise personnel, time and resource intensive. Groups attended four or five stations, spent approximately 20 minutes allowing sufficient time to identify key issues in complex labour scenarios.

Phase 3

To develop two identical, concurrent OSCE circuits and provide time for team building prior to commencement of the circuit.

Action

Extra faculty teaching staff were recruited as facilitators. This expanded teaching strategies and knowledge base of participants. Faculty facilitators also received feedback from observers.

Summary

The use of OSCE within inter-professional teams (ITOSCE) has been positively evaluated by faculty and students. Inter-professional learning between medical students and midwives enhances collaboration, breaks down professional boundaries and promotes teamwork in maternity services.

Chapter summary

- Identifying and analysing organizational culture is important in change management but extremely difficult to achieve because of its covert and implicit nature.
- Occupational groups in healthcare have different world views, histories, assumptions, values and language cultivated over many years.
- The most obvious evidence of culture are symbols which carry immense significance for group members.
- Medical culture has particular characteristics of status, privilege and expertise which may militate against multi-professional teamwork.

8

Organizational Learning and Analysis

Introduction

Chapters 4 and 7 discuss how organizations can begin with a small group of people, formed for a specific purpose to achieve certain defined goals, such as making a product or providing a service, and, over time and through growth and development of the product or service range, and requiring more people with a greater range of skills and knowledge, become progressively 'complex by design'.

With a small number of like-minded colleagues working together, decisions about work-based developments, job content, reward systems, performance measures, innovations and changes can be taken relatively easily through simple communication systems – there being little need for committees and detailed policies and procedures. As organizations expand there becomes a need to create systems dealing with human resources, finances, technical support, estates management, research and development, corporate governance and customer care, as well as regulatory and legislative demands and liaising with professional bodies, unions and shareholders. Thus the internal machinery develops to provide a robust administrative supporting structure enabling the efficient and effective functioning of the business environment. Over time, as these structures become larger, more complex and entrenched, so they solidify, administration becomes routinized, rigid and unmoveable and attracts the pejorative description 'bureaucracy'. Innovations become difficult to introduce and slow to take effect.

Since this text is aimed at frontline health professionals, most of whom will, by definition, work 'in the field' within large, bureaucratized organizations which are inherently resistant to change, and since current policy imperatives require those practitioners to be innovative and be 'the linchpin of change', working in 'new, more flexible ways' (DH, undated a), there is a notable dissonance between policy objectives, the nature of healthcare work and the organizational context. The only outcome of this will be practitioners' frustration and disillusionment; as Carroll and

Quijada (2004: ii16) note, 'Healthcare professionals have barely enough time and energy to cope with daily problems, leaving few resources for innovation and fundamental change'. One key reason for poor acceptance, take-up and diffusion of change implementation is the lack of sufficient attention to the organizational context (Fitzgerald et al., 2002).

Hence this chapter proposes means to analyse the organizational context through methods of enquiry, particularly around approaches to problem solving (Gorelick, 2005), and examines the significance of organizational learning as part of an overall strategy of implementing change. It therefore:

- outlines organizational knowledge required to initiate change;
- discusses the concepts of 'bureaucracy' and the 'learning organization' contrasting these with individual, team/group and organizational learning and revisiting aspects of organizational structure and culture;
- proposes a model which attempts to integrate individual, team and organizational learning;
- sets out a series of questions designed to encourage and enable health professionals to analyse their work context which can be used to 'defamiliarize' the local and the habitual;
- discusses the role of action research as a key method to promote organizational learning.

Through this, this chapter aims to consider the questions posed by Davies and Nutley (2000: 998) who ask: 'what does it mean to talk of an organization learning?' and 'can a hospital, general practice or health authority be said to learn?'

Organizational knowledge required to initiate change

Bauman argues that 'familiarity' through routine actions is the staunchest enemy of inquisitiveness and criticism and thus of change since problems and opportunities remain invisible. Inquisitiveness and criticism imply the ability to ask questions, employ analytical capabilities and learn from the findings:

Such questions make evident things into puzzles: they *defamiliarize* the familiar. Suddenly, the daily way of life must come under scrutiny. It now appears to be just one of the possible ways, not the one and only, not the 'natural' way of life. (Bauman, 1990: 15)

In analysing organizations, Hunt (1992) proposes two approaches. First, he discusses the 'analysis of variables' such as strategy, structure, leadership and culture, which have been raised in other chapters. Secondly, he suggests using a process method which concentrates on occurrences, events and problems, often termed 'triggers' (Paton and McCalman, 2000: 11) or critical incidents and examining how these are dealt with throughout the levels of the organization:

The most common analyses concentrate on the first and most elementary level – the individual actor. The second and more complex level involves groups of actors. This is the interpersonal level. Finally, the most complex and abstract level is to assess all the actors at once, as the organization. (Hunt, 1992: 154–5)

Many writers have identified key 'organizational level' knowledge for practitioners which affect the degree of success in initiating change. They argue those planning and initiating change must consider the following contextual factors:
Baldridge and Deal (1975: 1):

- A comprehensive organizational perspective and understanding of its subsystems.
- Strategies available to cause and support change.
- Personal and practical experience of the dynamics of change.

Salauroo and Burnes (1998: 452):

- The environment in which agents operate.
- The organization's 'internal cohesion'.
- Its leadership.
- The leaders' approach to change.

They conclude that those organizations which closely align these four elements are most successful at managing change.
Paton and McCalman (2000: 3):

- Circumstances surrounding a situation.
- Interaction of variables.
- Potential impact of associated variables.

They summarize that in change situations, a little knowledge can be dangerous and limited understanding catastrophic.
Ferlie and Shortell (2001: 282):

- Leadership at all levels.
- Pervasive culture that supports learning.
- An emphasis on the development of effective teams.
- Greater use of information technology.

Winyard (2003: 467):

- Establishing a strong case for change that 'signs up' those involved.
- Motivation: change is more effort in the short term than staying the same.
- Ensuring allocation of sufficient resources.

Though there are subtle differences, these writers all argue for a whole system multi-level approach, for deep knowledge and awareness of the organizational context, its culture and structural systems and the change focus itself. This indicates a model of 'insider action research' when members of an organization seek to 'inquire into the working of their organizational system in order to change something in it' (Coghlan, 2007: 336). Action research is an appropriate method of implementing change particularly where 'personal experience and knowledge of one's own system and job are a "pre-understanding" for the insider-researcher' (2007: 339). Furthermore, the processes, methods and focus of action research stress the importance of the group, rather than the individual in organizational change, and the centrality of experiential and reflective learning (Hendry, 1996) which has proved challenging within bureaucracies (DH, 2000b).

The limitations of bureaucracy

Originally the term 'bureaucracy' was applied to the body and workings of government administrative officials in Europe and came to epitomize the UK Civil Service as 'governors by profession, which is the essence and meaning of bureaucracy' (Mill, 1910: 245). Weber (1968) stressed the legitimized power of decision-making and 'rational' administrative efficiency in achieving goals through the principles of:

- Hierarchical structures of authority, supervision, specialization and departmentalization which channel communications through line management and co-ordinate decision-making – orders flowing down, responses flowing up.
- Clearly defined functionality governed by a binding, standardized set of written rules and procedures ensuring co-ordination, predictability and uniformity of operations which eliminates uncertainty and risk thus giving a rational-legal approach to problem-solving (see Table 7.1).
- The administrative separation of public and private affairs. Impersonal contact with clients (treated as 'cases') and subordinates designed to prevent emotional attachment distorting 'rational' decision-making.
- Division of labour through demarcated roles and functions, job description and salary; progression through the organization via merit or length of service.
- Employment of officials based on technical systems of selection and qualifications rather than familial or political patronage: rational equating of the role and function with qualifications is more important than the personal characteristics of the worker.

Giddens (1989: 277) explains that bureaucratic development is the 'only way of managing the administrative requirements of large-scale social systems' as it supposedly ensures criteria-based decisions, employee competence, and reduces corruption and kinship connections. Weber put it in these stark terms:

> Bureaucracy develops the more perfectly, the more it is 'dehumanised', the more completely it succeeds in eliminating from official business love, hatred and all purely personal ... and emotional elements which escape calculation. (Weber, 1968: 975)

Healthcare systems around the world are built on this dominant 'bureaucratic' model (Koeck, 1998) developing hugely cumbersome administrative structures. They are criticized for their multiple and often surplus functional tiers, written-based systems of communication, excessive administration, slow decision-making capabilities, lack of accountability and customer focus, command and control managerial approaches and centralizing systems (Baggott, 2004; Sheaff, 2005; Davidson and Peck, 2006). Chapter 1 rehearses the government's own reform plans designating the UK health system as '1940s, monolithic, top-down and centralized' (DH, 2002a: 3) while Howkins and Thornton (2002: 45) add the epithets 'hierarchical, authoritarian, closed, formal, tightly controlled … and directive'.

Weber (1968) termed bureaucracy an 'iron-cage' because of its tendency to become rule-bound and rigid; the condition where the 'bureaucracy' wields more power than the leaders or authority figures and where the adherence to rules and regulations become ends in themselves – to maintain the letter of the law becomes more important than to work within the spirit intended. Crozier (1964: 189) asserts that workers are unable to use individual initiative, managers are limited to controlling the application of rules, employees have no bargaining power over their leaders as they are 'totally deprived of initiative and completely controlled by the rules imposed'. In this way it is recognized that bureaucracies, such as hospitals and other healthcare organizations can stifle creativity and that staff are 'constrained by structures that limit development and innovation' (DH, 1999: 13).

The philosopher John Stuart Mill, writing in 1861, is even more critical:

> The disease which afflicts bureaucratic government … is routine. They perish by the immutability of their maxims; and … by the universal law that whatever becomes a routine loses its vital principle, and having no longer a mind acting within it, goes on revolving mechanically. (Mill, 1910: 246)

Koeck (1998: 1268) too criticizes the 'machine bureaucracy' which influences hospital thinking where 'all knowledge, responsibility, authority and power is vested at the top … from where it is delegated to lower levels' thus confirming the critical term 'top-down' so common in healthcare management. In this 'centralization of decisions' Crozier (1964: 189) adds that the power to make decisions and to interpret or change regulations or initiate new ones grows farther and farther away from 'the field' where practice is carried out. Therefore tension develops between encouraging innovation at the practitioner level and the perpetuation of procedures and routines; as Parkin (1997: 145) argues, when initiating change, forces maintaining the status quo tend to be stronger than forces for change. Mill argues that a bureaucracy 'bears down on the individuality of its more distinguished members' (1910: 246).

In widening criticism, Crozier (1964: 187) goes beyond the individual and sees a bureaucracy as 'an organization that cannot correct its behaviour by learning from its errors'. When a rule does not adequately deal with a 'case', rather than abandoning the rules, measures are taken to tighten them ensuring they are 'more complete, more precise, and more binding' than before. By using this description, Crozier introduces the idea of 'organizational learning' well before it became popular in the 1980s and 1990s (Burnes et al., 2003). It is a concept seen by organizational theorists as relevant to managing change and has close conceptual links with action research.

The centrality of learning

Though they are often the focus of change initiatives, solving everyday problems is not the same as changing organizations or situations nor can it be assumed that through solving a problem, individuals and organizations will learn. There need to be additional processes enacted to enable individuals to learn and to capture that learning and transform its diffusion beyond the immediate to the wider organizational environment.

In analysing the learning capacity of the NHS, the report *An Organization with a Memory* (DH, 2000b) focuses mainly on learning from failures and 'adverse events' and makes a distinction between passive learning, where lessons are identified but not put into practice, and active learning, where those lessons become embedded into an organization's culture and practices. This distinction is crucial in understanding why truly effective learning which produces change so often fails to take place.

The dilemma is whether learning from 'failure' focuses on the individual or the wider organizational system. The report claims the former dominates, seeing errors as resulting from individuals' lack of knowledge or skill, inattention to the task, forgetfulness and carelessness since this is more suited to the agenda of management and diverts attention away from the wider organizational systems which are harder to correct. Hence counter-measures are aimed at individuals rather than situations and systems and include disciplinary measures, individual training, writing more rules and procedures to guide individual behaviour or 'blaming, naming and shaming' (DH, 2000b: 20). So-called 'learning' is therefore premised negatively on avoiding mistakes rather than positively on developing and attaining excellence. This leads to practitioners becoming risk averse and prevents them from making even small changes in practice (Rushmer et al., 2004b) through fear of retribution in the face of failure (Attwood and Beer, 1988).

The report summarizes that the NHS does not learn actively or effectively from failures (where 'whistle-blowing' is evidence of a failure to learn), and it is '*par excellence* a passive learning organization' (DH, 2000b: 78). This situation persists: in reviewing 'complaints handling' the Healthcare Commission (2007) reports that systems still concentrate on following procedures rather than learning and assessing if care has changed as a result of a patient or client making a complaint.

In contrast, the 'systems approach' aims at wider data collection methods, clear communication and feedback channels and the creation of comprehensive programmes directed at individuals, teams, tasks, workplaces and institutions. It is these strategies that need to be implemented in order to develop 'learning cultures' particularly in large organizations (see Box 8.1).

Box 8.1

Overview

Thomas et al. (2005) report on a 'whole system' approach over three years in the UK to identify what organizational features support innovation in Primary Care Organizations (PCO). These PCOs are charged with empowering staff, through lifelong learning, to develop innovative services: they are large, mechanistic and bureaucratic; they process volumes of routine data; and are dysfunctional in radically changing environments. Learning organization theory and action research can be effective at supporting change but there is little knowledge about how complex bureaucracies can use and benefit from them.

Exploratory and fact-finding phase

PCO x 4 Study
Two PCOs were selected (one each from a deprived inner-city and suburban area) and two matched PCOs for comparison. Data were collected through:

- observation of meetings;
- analysis of strategic documents;
- interviews with 70 informants at project start and 2nd year – transcribed, analysed and validated.

Nurse Study

- Telephone interviews and focus group with 20 informants concerning organizational change and ability to innovate.

Financial Study

- Interviews with six finance directors/managers from four PCOs.

London Study

- 2000 – Data from 63 organizations regarding organizational development strategies.
- 2001 – Purposive sample interviewed regarding progress.
- 2002 – 32 PCO chief executives questioned and six telephone interviews.

Decision and action phase

Facilitators helped staff 'make sense' of data and changes.

Annual conferences were scheduled where participants (25 in 2000; 70 in 2001; 41 in 2002) could debate the meaning of data and design the next phase of project. Stakeholders were enthusiastic about organizational learning and the role of action research in helping to understand learning and change.

Features associated with organizational capacity for learning

1 High quality leadership, understandable corporate governance, a capacity for reflection and intention to work with principles of organizational learning.

---

2   External facilitation was useful. Facilitators observed 13 sub-committees in one PCO leading to action which developed committee chairs and cross-committee representation to connect organizational learning.

3   Opportunities for reflection at all organizational levels through sub-committee cross-representation enabled 'giving voice' to employees.

4   Both clinicians and managers were needed with a leadership style which encouraged participation with a 'learning – not blaming – culture' (Thomas et al., 2005: 315).

5   Timing of an initiative was an important determinant of success.

Features related to low morale

1   Pace of policy implementation limited capacity for reflection.

2   Staff experience and infrastructure was inadequate to manage scale of change.

3   Finance limited organizational development.

Summary

The PCOs tried to overcome a 'bureaucratising tendency' (Thomas et al., 2005: 316) through bottom-up reflection and facilitation to promote innovation, change and learning. However, most 'innovations' were adaptations of existing ideas. The only true 'innovation' was the 'whole-system' cross-committee learning which showed that incremental experiential learning translated into organization-wide intelligence.

Hendry (1996) argues that learning theory should be central to the creation and development of learning cultures. As innovation and continuous improvement become increasingly important, and people are recognized as the principal source of competitive advantage, Hendry argues that organizations need to look at how far they function as learning cultures. Therefore discovering and understanding the linkages integrating individual, team and organizational learning become vital in the change management process.

The learning organization

Though not a new concept, interest in 'organizational' as opposed to 'individual' learning in organizational theory has burgeoned in the last 20 years and is an important concept within the broad sweep of change management literature. However, like many of the concepts drawn on in this text, its existence lacks empirical evidence, particularly in the public sector (Betts and Holden, 2003); its meaning is disputed by the many theorists claiming a stake in its use and it is difficult to attain (Edge and Laiken, 2002). Applying the term 'competence' as a combination of knowledge, technical and performance management skills, Dunphy et al. (1997: 236) see a learning organization as one 'which develops and maintains competencies both to perform and to change in order to maintain or improve performance'. Hunt (1992) takes a 'problem-centred view' and believes a learning organization is characterized by involvement of all employees in identifying and solving problems, and enables them continuously to experiment, improve and increase their capacity to deliver.

Some writers note the difference between a 'learning organization' as a noun describing a type of organization and an aspirational goal, an end state that can be achieved (which Burnes et al. (2003) claim few, if any, reach) and 'organizational learning' as a verb describing the processes of, and attempts by, organizations to learn (Burnes et al., 2003; Gorelick, 2005). With few criteria to define the former, Burnes et al. (2003) argue the latter, more sceptical position is preferable. Gorelick (2005: 384) prefers to see them co-existing but poses the question that if organizational learning is a continuous cycle then an organization cannot arrive at a point of being 'a learning organization'. In contrast, Burnes et al. (2003: 454) state that a 'learning organization is the highest state of organizational learning' where it has achieved the 'ability to transform itself continuously through the development and involvement of all its members'.

Rowden (2001: 15–16) outlines four main characteristics of learning organizations:

- Constant readiness: staff are prepared for continuous change in general, not a specific change. This occurs through being attuned to the environment and willing to question fundamental ways of acting.
- Continual planning: flexible plans are fully shared and embraced by the entire organization. 'Revision' is more important than 'vision'.
- Improvised implementation: plans are not executed by numbers, improvisation and experimentation are encouraged. Successes are reinforced and structures modified.
- Action learning: the learning organization takes action, reflects on results and adjusts as it progresses.

Learning: individual → group → organization

Many writers take a dyadic approach considering only the individual and the organizational levels (Lipshitz and Popper, 2000), omitting vital learning at the group or team level.

Bohmer and Edmonson (2001) argue that for hospitals to achieve their goals and improve, learning must occur at the individual, group and organizational levels but that the historical and current focus, particularly within medicine, is with the individual practitioner. Here, learning is achieved through 'correcting' poor practice through learning from mistakes, employing repetitive practice and close adherence to clinical guidelines reflecting Taylorist ideas of the 'one best way'.

Individual level

There is insufficient space to outline the many and varied theories of learning which derive from the behavioural, cognitive, humanistic and social learning perspectives. The salient aspects which relate to change management are developed as strategies in Chapter 11.

Individual learning is the principal and enduring focus of almost all educational programmes (Betts and Holden, 2003) which tend to be structured and linear and focus on detecting and rectifying faults or misconceptions. Learning is therefore seen through a 'behaviourist' lens and as a stimulus–response mechanism where it is defined as 'relatively permanent change in behaviour occurring as a result of experience or practice' (Hilgard and Atkinson, 1967: 270). This equates broadly to the behavioural definitions applied to organizational learning above. Lewin (1942/1997: 216) sees learning more broadly in practical terms of 'doing something better than before' and distinguishes

- change in cognitive structure (knowledge);
- change in motivation;
- change in group belongingness or ideology (culture).

A definition which can be applied equally to individuals, teams and organizations is to define learning as 'the process whereby knowledge is created through the transformation of experience' (Kolb, 1984: 38).

In general, experience in healthcare suggests that individuals may learn from their mistakes but others around them often fail to do so (DH, 2000b), a point noted by Bohmer and Edmonson (2001) who claim that practitioners are often uncomfortable discussing errors with colleagues. This focus on the individual makes it harder for systems to learn and spread the impact of incidents beyond their immediate environment (DH, 2000b).

Simons (2002), for example, discusses an action research project which aims to improve pain management in children. An educational programme was targeted at nurses who identified that pain control was not always managed appropriately in their work areas. They benefited as individuals but appeared powerless to translate their learning to their units or across professional boundaries to create wider organizational learning in an important area of paediatrics that is poorly understood:

> The nurses felt there was room for improvement in the management of pain in their areas … and expressed frustration with both nursing and medical colleagues and suggested that their colleagues should all attend … to improve their practice. (Simons, 2002: 113–14)

Indeed, Chan's (2003) survey of 198 respondents in an Australian hospital claims individual learning was not significantly related to any of the organizational learning attributes but was significantly related to team learning. Betts and Holden (2003) report that participants' lack of power in a local authority prevented them from applying their learning in the workplace. Rushmer et al. (2004b) also note that knowledge generated through experience is seldom captured so when staff leave or retire their knowledge leaves with them. Successful outcomes for individual learning do not guarantee successful outcomes in organizational learning.

The common practice of the annual individual performance appraisal is seen as contributing negatively to both team and organizational learning. Padaki (2002) claims organizational learning is the product of the interactivity of all the parts. Treating parts separately through individual appraisals illustrates the fallacy of the mechanistic approach leading to sub-optimal learning of the system.

Group or team level

Rather than applying the term 'learning organization', Hendry analyses the level between the individual and the organization as 'communities of practice' which are the relationships people create and develop to solve problems in practice:

> People share tacit knowledge and through dialogue bring this to the surface; they exchange ideas about work practice and experiment with new methods and ideas; they engage in discussions which affirm or modify theories in use; they innovate new problem-solving routines and simultaneously manage and repair the social context. In other words, they engage in experiential learning, develop and refine cognitive structures and engage in culture formation. (Hendry, 1996: 628)

Group or team learning is therefore seen as occurring when there is constant dialogue and feedback which involves people in deep inquiry (Yeo, 2006) and, whereas individual learning is a cognitive and reflective process (Betts and Holden, 2003), team and organizational learning is embedded in social processes. Hendry then develops this further using action research as the key method of learning within communities of practice:

> How then does 'learning' take place? Action research, as a methodology that focuses on groups to effect change, and the emerging concept of communities-of-practice both point to the key role of groups, their tacit knowledge, experiential learning, and the location of learning in a socialization process as core elements. (Hendry, 1996: 626)

This is an approach taken up by Lathlean and le May (2002) who describe four action research projects undertaken in healthcare and see communities of practice as effective means of developing inter-agency working which promote partnerships and positively influence service design and delivery.

Bohmer and Edmonson (2001) argue that though the team should be the fundamental unit of learning in complex organizations, team learning does not happen naturally. Rather it has to be managed. It is a community activity which is deliberate and dynamic (Benoit and Mackensie, 1994). This is because of the unique make-up of different teams, their collective experience, their interactions and dynamic culture. Where translating individual learning into organizational learning is affected by power structures and dynamics, the collective force of team learning may ameliorate these limitations. Team learning is dependent on cultural aspects, the quality of relationships and interaction between group members and group leadership (Lipshitz and Popper, 2000). Teams therefore learn differently and at different speeds. Timpson (1998) also cautions that not all members are willing to participate in active learning and embrace the added responsibilities that go along with it. Strategies which focus on change through team learning are developed in Chapter 11.

Organization level

Bohmer and Edmonson (2001: 32) define organizational learning as 'a process of improving organizational actions through acquiring and developing new knowledge and capabilities'. Furthermore, they argue that an organization is said to have learnt, 'when its actions have changed' as a result of new knowledge and insight.

The connections and differences between individual learning and organizational learning are vigorously debated but not always with clarity. For example, Dunphy et al. (1997: 232) claim that current contributions to the debate 'focused on individual learning rather than organizational learning'. Benoit and Mackensie (1994: 26) criticize theorists' approaches if they 'view organizational learning as an outcome of individuals in the organization, rather than an outcome of the organization itself'. Amitay et al. (2005: 57) argue that confusion around organizational learning stems from treating individual-level learning and organizational-level learning as 'one and the same'. In an opposing view, Bruce and Wyman (1998: 220) reiterate that organizations are 'groups of people working together to achieve a common purpose'. Without individuals organizations would not exist; they would be unable to communicate, take strategic actions, make mistakes or solve problems. Bruce and Wyman further assert:

> Organizations do not really change, only the people in them do. If the people do not change … then the organization cannot really change. If the people in the organization do not learn, the organization does not learn either. (Bruce and Wyman, 1998: 15–16)

Hunt (1992: 135) also argues that analysis at the organizational level is risky and can lead to the 'trap of suggesting that the [organization] is a living entity with a life independent of the people in it'. Lipshitz and Popper (2000) therefore argue that organizational learning must be treated metaphorically since giving organizations human-like qualities of perceiving, reasoning and remembering is problematic. Organizational learning can therefore be seen as a system of actions and processes enabling an organization to continually integrate information, knowledge and experiences gained from internal and external sources, into ways and means of successfully changing and adapting. This indicates clear connective processes acting between and within individuals, groups and organizations.

Proposal of a model connecting individual, group and organizational learning

Figure 8.1 is developed from the management model in Figure 4.1 and the 'Dynamic model of change' in Figure 6.4. Its development employs a similar approach deriving the major concepts from the literature, research and practice. The 'influencing factors' on the left are identified as the most relevant contributors to organizational learning and are derived from Figure 4.1. The cyclic 'process approach to learning' on the right reflects the approach used in the dynamic model of change in Figure 6.4 and the action

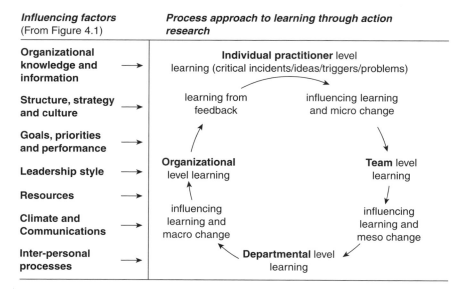

Figure 8.1 Dynamic model for organizational learning through action research

Source: developed from Parkin (1999a)

research process in Figure 6.5. Furthermore, it aims to integrate the 'levels of aggregation' described by Coghlan and Casey (2001: 679) and De Loo (2002), including not only the levels of analysis discussed above but an intermediate 'interdepartmental' level.

The contribution to organizational learning works through the 'interlevel dynamics such as the impact the individual has on the team and vice versa, the team on other teams, and the organization on individuals, teams and on the interdepartmental group and vice versa' (Coghlan and Casey, 2001: 679). Chan (2003) sees the collective intelligence of teams as a precursor to organizational learning:

> Hospital staff might not be learning directly from individual members but through teams, and a team learns from individual members and the knowledge gained transpires to organizational level. (Chan, 2003: 229–30)

Lipshitz and Popper (2000) discuss 'organizational learning mechanisms' where the experiences of individual members are analysed and shared by member groups (teams) then, through distribution of 'lessons learnt' or changes in standard procedures, become the property of the entire organization.

In the action research study in Box 8.1, Thomas et al. (2005) argue that PAR introduced the idea of a research community where people of different backgrounds work together over a research question. They report that it is the collective knowledge and experience of the various individual and complementary perspectives which are particularly valuable in learning especially when complex or contested phenomena are involved. Learning is not simply the sum of the individuals' knowledge (Padaki, 2002; Rushmer et al., 2004b), rather it is the knowledge, skills and experiences held 'collectively and in common' by the group (Rushmer et al., 2004c: 389).

Action research and organizational analysis

Coughlan and Coghlan (2002: 225) claim that researchers need not only a broad view of how the formal and technical sub-systems work but also the informal 'people' sub-systems. Working with organizational systems requires an ability to work with dynamic complexity which has a political dimension. Coghlan and Casey suggest that carrying out action research is both political and subversive as it examines issues, incites action, endorses democratic participation and emphasizes questioning which are all threatening to individuals, teams and organizational norms:

> In order that individual learning is aggregated into organizational learning, action researchers need to work effectively at all four levels ... with individuals, teams, across the interdepartmental group and organization. This is critical to bridging the wide gap that exists between individual and organizational learning. (Coghlan and Casey, 2001: 679–80)

Livesey and Challender (2002) argue that if organizational learning is to be the result of action research, then the rationale for the intervention must be owned by those in the problem situation. Rushmer et al. (2004b) emphasize that organizational learning (and action research) is not just about solving problems but also improving situations before problems emerge.

Asking questions and diagnosing problems

Coghlan and Casey (2001: 678) argue that of central importance to action researchers is the need to gather data, stimuli and perceptions as part of the 'diagnosing' phase (see 'pre-plan' stage in Figure 4.1; Figure 2.1). The subsequent 'sense-making process' indicates the need for them to have good organizational and analytical capabilities which come through asking questions about issues and problems in practice. However, Beer and Eisenstat (1996: 600) claim that in many organizations there is a low level of competence in developing an 'inquiring dialogue' which inhibits the identification of the root causes of problems and potential solutions.

Asking questions

Although these questions fall under the overall heading of 'organizational analysis' they mirror the 'Exploratory/Diagnostic/Fact finding phase' of the action research process outlined in Chapter 2 and have been developed from Hunt (1992: 268), Hart and Bond (1995: 186–90), Parkin (1997: 143) and Bruce and Wyman (1998).

Questions are important but unsettling: they intrude as uninvited guests; they act as meddlesome strangers; they disturb the comfortable way of life; they turn things that were once obvious into puzzles; they defamiliarize the familiar (Bauman, 1990); and they surface normally hidden issues which may be threatening or embarrassing (Beer and Eisenstat, 1996).

1 What (exactly) is the trigger/problem/issue/change focus?

- Is this the first 'noticing' or has it been noticed but ignored before and is it recurring?
- How widespread is the problem, how many people are involved and who and what does it affect?
- Is the problem: geographical, social, cultural, technical, strategic?
- What solutions have been attempted, with what result?
- If they failed, why?
- Why is it important to do something about it?
- Is there agreement about the problem and solutions?

Coghlan and Casey (2001: 678) argue that it is important to uncover the issues that are viewed by staff as major and which require attention. Beer and Eisenstat (1996) note that where there is no agreed diagnosis, neither a common vision of a future state nor a coherent intervention can be negotiated.

2 What are the causes of the problem/s?

Here analysis is developed through the processes of:

- Noticing – identifying, collecting and monitoring data.
- Interpreting – assessing the data and determining, if possible, potential causes.
- Incorporating – relating interpretations to the goals and values of the organization.

In the action research example in Box 3.2 (Mitchell et al., 2005), the trigger was the discovery of incorrect manual handling procedures through poor knowledge and understanding. The values underpinning change were to provide high quality care to patients and promote multi-disciplinary working between nurses and physiotherapists.

3 What are the consequences of not addressing the problem?

Wallis and Tyson indicate how staff in a Haematology-Oncology Day Unit (HODU) gradually became aware of a developing problem and noted the negative ramifications, particularly quality of patient care, if it was not addressed:

> The staff of one HODU became aware that the increasing diversification of the patients being treated in the unit was causing a rise in the demand for service. This in turn was causing delays for patients and a possible reduction in the standard of care provided. The

charge nurse was receiving more patient complaints … nurses were expressing their concerns about the level of care they were able to provide. There were concerns about patient waiting lists, the time patients had to wait on treatment days, patient symptom management, patient education, and the identification and management of chemotherapy complications. (Wallis and Tyson, 2003: 75–6)

These questions reflect Plsek and Wilson's (2001) concept of 'direction-pointing'. Precise problem identification in these cases is not simple or straightforward. Lippitt et al. (1958) state that as data are collected and analysed, the problem which originally seemed simple and bounded is likely to take on the appearance of an intricate, many-faceted difficulty. Hart and Bond (1995) imply that a problem for one group may not be seen as a problem for another which has implications for problem ownership (Reed, 2005).

4 What is the climate of opinion?

- Can the situation be solved or improved?
- Does the initiative conflict with other priorities?
- Will it improve things for the:
  - patient/client;
  - individual practitioner;
  - team;
  - organization as a whole.

The study in Box 8.2 shows that staff in the rehabilitation team were keen to critically examine their practice, introduce innovations and work collectively, extending to visiting and sharing practice with an external unit.

Box 8.2

Overview

Bennett (1998) reports on the early stages of a project to focus the activity and increase collaboration within a multi-disciplinary rehabilitation team in a general hospital in the UK.

Setting

The large team comprised nursing, physiotherapy, occupational, communication, art and music therapy, medicine, psychology and social work groups. The weekly ward round was inefficient due to lack of focus and team discipline and previous attempts at improving effectiveness and collaboration had failed:

- Introduction of new patient record system fell into disuse after a few weeks.
- Introduction of 'generic rehabilitation assistant' failed to gain support.
- Actions agreed following team building workshops stopped.

(Continued)

(Continued)

Trigger

An opportunity arose to develop 'patient-centred goal planning' (P-CGP) which the team felt could resolve problems of focus and collaboration and improve patient care. Action research offered a more appropriate framework for involvement and systematic and evolutionary change. P-CGP was crucial for motivation and successful rehabilitation from brain injury but presented a challenge to therapists who needed to work together to avoid role duplication.

Planning and action phase

Five team members attended a workshop provided by an out-of-region Rehabilitation Centre which had introduced and published on P-CGP.

- Team meeting convened to feedback and decide action.
- Generated questions, discussion, checking for areas of consensus and conflict.
- Agreement to pursue P-CGP.
- Agreement on auditing process.

Second phase

- Further staff meetings to examine detail of P-CGP.
- Practised setting aims, objectives and targets.
- Agreed to use new documentation with all new admissions.
- Reviewed each patient case two weeks post admission.
- To generate confidence, mock case reviews were run using new documentation enabling the team to learn from mistakes and make improvements.

Third phase

Second delegation sent to out-of-area Rehabilitation Centre for further reconnaissance.

- Meeting held to clarify learning needs.
- On return, further meetings clarified process of goal planning.
- Piloting of P-CGP with 10 consecutive patients agreed.

Summary

Through discussion of published work, attendance at workshops and using documentation of the Rehabilitation Centre, action research is shown to be generalizable where there are shared theories, goals and values especially where patient care is central.

Introducing a change through the exploration of P-CGP has been straightforward and unproblematic 'primarily facilitated by the use of action research' (Bennett, 1998: 231).

Baldridge and Deal (1975) argue that ultimately the benefit to the client is the only goal worth fighting for and this has been reflected in the action research studies identified in this text. Furthermore Lippitt et al. (1958) note that no situation is ever static; improvements are always possible provided that there is agreement on how these are defined. The organization's statement of values and mission will indicate a project's potential acceptance by senior management. Projects which are congruent with an organization's values or increase its performance are more likely to be supported and resourced (Buchanan et al., 2005).

5 Who are the major stakeholders?

From this can be ascertained who will help and who will hinder development and progress? Whose support is vital and whose opinion can be disregarded? Who acts as gatekeepers to open and close doors? It reflects Plsek and Wilson's (2001) concept of 'gaining permission'. Hart and Bond (1995) suggest subsequent questions will emerge:

- What are the major stakeholders' positions?
- What is their perspective on the problem?
- How much power do they hold?
- Is there open access to data?

These positions should be evaluated as often practitioners do not have enough power and influence in the system to implement change (Parkin, 1997). Bennett (1998) recalls how an earlier initiative of introducing a 'generic' rehabilitation worker combining nursing, physiotherapy and occupational therapy support roles failed through lack of managerial support (Box 8.2).

Further questions include:

- How much freedom is there in decision-making?
- What is the stakeholder's strength of control?

In their action research project to introduce Nurse Practitioners to carry out work normally undertaken by GPs, Livesey and Challender (2002) found tensions between the GPs, who wanted their problems solved, the 'client' (the head of Primary Care Services (PCS)), who wanted to maintain the service contract and the university providing the researcher who wanted to generate publications. These power dynamics made it difficult to engage the parties in meaningful discussions about the problem. Once Livesey (as the researcher/problem solver) grasped this she claims: 'The positional power held by that individual (the head of PCS) to facilitate the problem solving process is now seen to be critical in managing politics which were not the responsibility of the problem solver' (Livesey and Challender, 2002: 174). Nevertheless, she found moving and maintaining the stakeholders in the same direction a major distraction from the task.

6 What will it cost and who will pay?

Implementing change involves using extra resources. These may have cost implications which were not budgeted for. In the majority of studies identified in this text, services are improved, evaluated and developed through the existing human, material, financial and technological resources within the organization. Good practice implies that an action plan should include a budget covering:

- human resource costs
- additional skills, knowledge or IT resources
- space and equipment costs.

In addition to the above resources, estimates should address design costs, time-span of the project and costs of the main participants if absent from their normal work roles (see Box 8.2). Practitioners should be aware of development costs, particularly if a new service is proposed, and engage in cost control and monitor expenditure. Where cost benefits and cost-effectiveness can be obtained from similar examples, these can be used for benchmark estimates. Proposals for increasing client satisfaction should also be outlined.

7 Is the change superficial or fundamental?

Coghlan and Brannick (2001) see modern organizations as centres of politics, infighting, cliques and political factions; a stark contrast, they claim, to the impersonal formal rational image portrayed by Weber's 'ideal type'. Where change is featured, especially the control, allocation and distribution of resources, power politics, in the shape of resistance and conflict can emerge with force. Parkin (1997) suggests it is therefore worth considering all change as being fundamental to some faction and to proceed with caution:

> There are fundamental territorial issues which should be recognized, ownership of knowledge, space, time, equipment and resources. They indicate professional values and issues of power and status and the control of one individual or group over others and hence involve beliefs and values. It is therefore worth considering all change as being fundamental to some person or group. (Parkin, 1997: 146)

These issues can create tensions, resistance and conflict which are examined further in Chapters 9 and 10.

The force field analytical tool

A basic and useful tool, the 'force field analysis' can assist the examination of these driving and restraining forces in any situation. Apart from being integral to Lewin's planned approach to change, this simple device can be used to:

- map out, illustrate and understand where power lies
- assess the relative strength of forces
- assess how they influence the actions of individuals and groups in change situations
- provide an opportunity to involve other participants in the change process.

Table 8.1   Force field analysis: example of a nurse implementing a wound assessment chart into the assessment process

Driving Forces – Strength/Level			Restraining Forces – Strength/Level	
Trust standard already set	5L	➤ ◄	Standard not owned by group	5M
Support from tissue viability team	5M	➤ ◄	Adds more work	5M
General interest from team	3H	➤ ◄	Training input required	3M
Change will encourage learning	3H	➤ ◄	Time constraints	3L
Evidence it improves care	5L	➤ ◄	Disputed value	1H

Scoring:
Numbers = **Strength** of forces:
1 = low; 3 = medium; 5 = high
Letters = How **easily** forces can be influenced by change agents:
H = high; M = medium; L = low

Though Figure 6.1 shows broad concepts, in reality, more detailed and specific forces can be identified, including those of powerful leaders and managers (see Table 8.1). Lewin (1947/1997: 320) suggests that 'diminishing the opposing forces' produces less tension and resistance than increasing forces for change and that consequently the former, though counterintuitive, is a more effective change strategy.

Coghlan and Casey (2001: 676) set out some of the challenges to researchers examining their own organizations. They may find it difficult to obtain data if they have to 'cross departmental, functional, hierarchical boundaries'. As an 'insider' they may be denied deeper access. Knowledge is both powerful and political and the degree to which this is shared will have an effect on outcomes. Practitioners therefore require the skills of justifying, influencing and negotiating, and need to consider the impact of healthcare politics on the process of change.

Conclusion

Whatever term is used, organizational learning signifies important concepts within change efforts. De Loo (2002) claims that it may be impossible to describe precisely the relationship between individual and organizational learning. Where practitioners engage in their own, or preferably collective, analysis and questioning of their organizational systems to ascertain where problems and change opportunities lie; where there are group- and team-wide initiatives; where problems and opportunities become agreed and owned by the group and the pool of potential solutions, knowledge and experience is expanded and risk of mistakes and failure is reduced and dispersed, only in these situations can initiatives become 'bottom-up' and counter the regulatory and binding tendencies of bureaucracies.

Chapter summary

- Bureaucratic hierarchies operate within rigid rules and procedures to appear rational and reduce risk.
- Working within rules and procedures stifles practitioner innovation through conformity and defensive routines.
- Working outside rules and procedures stifles practitioner innovation through fear of failure and retribution.
- Focusing on individual learning limits the organization's capacity to learn.
- Cultivating team-level learning offers a more robust model for knowledge diffusion and organizational learning.

9

Reactions to Change 1: Resistance

Introduction

Thus far this text has promoted the view that if implementing change in healthcare improves the quality of services to patients and clients and creates and develops individual, team and organizational learning then it should be seen as positive and consequently welcomed by staff. However, acceptance of a change and the concomitant disruption and learning is an intensely personal judgement taken by individuals, usually working in groups or teams, and influenced by a wide range of emotional, psychological, social, political and technical factors. Many of these influences may remain hidden from both practitioners themselves and their managers, but Kotter (1990) claims that reactions to change are often influenced through a personal assessment of its potential impact employing the central but self-serving question 'how will this affect me?'

Traditionally, resistance is defined where change implementers perceive a difficulty in having their ideas accepted or the change is thwarted or sabotaged by others. It is usually seen as negative and as 'the enemy of change' (Waddell and Sohal, 1998: 544). Hence, Balfour and Clarke (2001: 45) argue that the biggest 'hurdle to cross' when considering an innovation is 'overcoming' resistance.

Its literal meaning is from the Latin '*resistere*', to 'make a stand against' and synonyms range in strength from 'non-cooperation', 'confrontation' and 'struggle', to 'conflict', 'fight' and 'battle' so its negative subtext seems appropriate. Its antonym is 'surrender' signifying giving up through weakness or the inability to organize sufficient forces to win. Furthermore, in the current achievement-oriented climate of public-sector work, failing or losing are politically and socially stigmatized positions to be avoided. When progress in organizational life is concerned with 'winning' (Buchanan and Badham, 1999), and winners can become heroes and champions it is easy to see how losing (either by change agents or 'resistors') can affect reputations and future prospects and opportunities.

Giangreco and Peccei (2005) note that resistance takes many forms and distinguish between explicit protests and collective resistance such as strikes and industrial action with the more covert, subtle and passive forms of 'dissent' or 'reluctance' such as failure to support change or engage in pro-change behaviour.

Noting the limitations of language and the need for a 'multidimensional' view of resistance (Piderit, 2000; Oreg, 2006), it is more instructive to use neutral terminology such as 'reactions' or 'responses' to change. This may assist in focusing on both the content and outcomes of change and the processes of implementation, and move beyond a limiting 'individualized' conception of resistance to a wider, more systemic view.

Nevertheless, beginning with early studies relating to change (Coch and French, 1947; Lewin, 1947/1997), understanding and managing reactions emerge as key and enduring themes (Elsey and Lathlean, 2006) and need to be seriously considered in order for an organization to benefit from change initiatives (Pardo del Val and Martinez Fuentes, 2003).

This chapter therefore discusses:

- The nature and changing perspectives of resistance.
- Understanding the context of reactions to change.
- Individual, group and organizational reactions.
- Action research as a strategy for management.

The chapter is illustrated by two action research studies (Waterson, 2000; Reed, 2005) which recount and analyse why staff in health and social care settings react negatively to the introduction of new ways of working.

Nature of resistance

As models of change are re-examined and reassessed through research, the literature on 'resistance to change' is being re-evaluated and can appear contradictory and confusing. Following an extensive literature review, Dent and Powley (2002) assert that there is no commonly held definition of resistance nor an accepted, validated scale for its measurement (Giangreco and Peccei, 2005). The continuum of perspectives extends from Dent and Goldberg's (1999: 26) statement that 'we assert ... that people do *not* resist change' to Krantz's (1999: 43) direct repost to their view stating 'I, for one, believe that people at all levels of organizational life *do* resist change'.

Dent and Goldberg (1999) argue that the current concept of resistance and the expectation that people will resist change arises from a 'bankrupt' mental model which has taken on universal acceptance as an unchallenged 'fact'. In doing so it distorts the implementation process causing organizations to engage in unnecessary and unproductive actions to 'correct' or 'overcome' it. They suggest that the term should be dispensed with and more useful and appropriate models found to describe what it has come to mean. These shifting orientations are now discussed.

The original view

The original conception of resistance can be found in Lewin's (1947/1997: 309) discussion of group dynamics under the heading 'Constancy and Resistance to Change'. Here he discusses the output of a small group working in equilibrium (constancy): 'no individual leaves or joins … no friction occurs … unchanged level of production … the same conditions lead to the same effect' (1947/1997: 309). He then describes the difference if a member is absent: 'If, in spite of such changes in the group … production is kept at the same level, then one can speak of "resistance" to change the rate of production'.

In other words the group worked to 'counteract' the effects of the change – they 'resisted' the 'changes' to their work rate by working harder to ensure their output did not fall. Importantly both the source of change and their reaction (resistance) were located within the system of work rather than in worker's minds or emotions. In the classic study on worker participation and resistance, Coch and French (1947) also outline the influence of systemic 'force fields' (see Figure 6.1). In the Harwood factory improvements to worker output were achieved using action research. The main forces acting in a 'downward' direction (resistance) were found to be:

- difficulty of the job;
- avoidance of strain (overwork);
- group pressure to restrict production.

The forces acting in an 'upward' direction were:

- achieving the 'standard production' target (perceived success);
- pressures of management supervision (this was 'encouragement' rather than 'coercion');
- group pressure of competition.

Coch and French (1947: 529) summarize that the most important force affecting work was 'the standard set by the group' (what would now be called group culture) which affected all group members and, they claim, could be more powerful than any force induced by management. Reactions to change were found to be a 'complex affair' relating to the actual work, the group dynamics, the standards set and relationship with managers. Overall they report that performance and efficiency were directly proportional to levels of worker participation, and that rates of turnover and aggression were inversely proportional to the amount of participation. Thus, resistance was appreciated as being diffused throughout the production systems and processes. An example is the greater 'resistance' imposed as workers come closer to reaching a high standard. A contemporary representation would be an athlete attempting to break a world track-record; there are a number of collateral factors to harmonize affecting the likelihood of success, including fitness levels, training schedules, mental attitude, competitive spirit, competitor support, venue, climate, wind speed, track surface and design of running shoes, all of which act collectively as 'resistors' to achievement.

The traditional view

Krantz (1999: 42–3) argues that since Lewin's time the concept of resistance to change has been transformed into 'a not-so-disguised way of blaming the less powerful for unsatisfactory results of change efforts' and has been 'distorted and used to provide managers with an easy, blame-shifting explanation for a far more complex reality'. Dent and Powley (2002) claim that change failures are now attributed to worker resistance as a convenient scapegoat absolving managers from culpability. Giangreco and Peccei (2005) note that studies of resistance have traditionally been taken from the change agents' perspective rather than the clients', casting it negatively as a sign of failure and the resistant worker as 'subversive' (Waddell and Sohal, 1998: 543) and an 'obstacle' (Piderit, 2000: 784). Dent and Goldberg (1999) argue that current management texts create the expectation of resistance and treat it as a psychological concept located solely within the individual. Thus Coghlan claims: 'Resistance is a label generally applied by managers and consultants to the perceived behaviour of organization members who seem unwilling to accept or help implement an organizational change' (1993: 10).

In an attempt to capture the complexity of resistance Piderit (2000) and Oreg (2006: 76) define it as 'a tri-dimensional attitude towards change which includes affective, behavioural and cognitive components':

- 'Affective' concerns individuals' emotions (fear, anxiety).
- 'Behavioural' involves taking or planning intentional action (complaining, inciting others).
- 'Cognitive' concerns individuals' thoughts (is it necessary or beneficial?).

Piderit (2000) explains that individuals' responses may lie anywhere along the continuum of each dimension ranging between extreme positives and negatives. She also outlines that the separate dimensions allow for different reactions along different dimensions. This means that someone can show 'ambivalence' about change where a positive cognitive response (this change is good for the department) may conflict with a negative emotional response (I don't want to lose my role). Behavioural ambivalence may exhibit in an individual through covert opposition (by sending anonymous feedback comments) whilst demonstrating public support through fear of management retribution.

Pardo del Val and Martinez Fuentes (2003: 149) and Hunt (1992: 291) define resistance as 'any conduct which attempts to preserve the status quo' in the face of pressures or actions to alter it. Hunt argues that resistance is the most frequently cited reason for failure in organizational change and is linked with feelings of fear, uncertainty and a perceived loss of control.

Other writers disagree: Kegan and Lahey (2001: 85) state that 'resistance to change does not reflect opposition, nor is it the result of inertia', rather people display a 'personal immunity to change' (see below).

Ford et al. (2002) note that when resistance is objectified to the individual, management strategies focus on changing those individuals rather than wider systems. This not only creates more resistance but is far removed from Lewin's original conception that resistance is diffused throughout a system.

The emerging view

Giangreco and Peccei (2005) note that recently a more objective and positive approach to resistance is being taken. Pardo del Val and Martinez Fuentes (2003) argue that since change in organizations is not always beneficial, so attempts to avoid change through inertia and resistance cannot necessarily be seen as negative. Others point to the positive aspects of resistance. Lamb and Cox (1999) argue that resistance to change is healthy and that without real questioning and scepticism it is unlikely that an organization can progress to a productive stage of learning and working in any new structure. Mabin et al. (2001) argue that resistance is better than apathy as it avoids group-think and provides more alternatives from more people.

Perren and Megginson (1996: 24) suggest that the prevailing negative view of resistance to change may be wrong and that far from being a hindrance it can actually be a benefit to an organization and should be encouraged. They claim at best, such resistance could be seen as a 'natural' survival mechanism within organizations that 'tests, adapts and sometimes stops decisions by fallible and often ill-informed senior managers'. This is because resistors may have a more detailed understanding of the organizational consequences than those driving change. Waddell and Sohal (1998) argue that resistance plays a crucial role in highlighting aspects of change that may be inappropriate, badly thought through or plain wrong. In this way resistance creates energy and, through following a parliamentary model of scrutiny and 'devils advocacy', becomes a trigger to search for alternatives. Thus resistance itself becomes a springboard for innovation.

Change content or change process?

Further contentions emerge: Giangreco and Peccei (2005: 1817) state that two key factors, the 'content of change' and the 'implementation process' have 'received the greatest emphasis and attention in the literature' in affecting resistance. Oreg (2006: 78) disputes this claiming that the literature 'does not distinguish between the two types of reactions: reactions to change outcomes and reactions to the change process'.

Content

From a 'content' or outcomes perspective, Waddell and Sohal (1998) propose that people resist the uncertainties that change foreshadows.

Dent and Goldberg (1999) agree that people will assess the degree that change affects factors such as loss of status, pay, comfort and social relationships through a 'cost–benefit analysis' (Giangreco and Peccei, 2005) including how potential changes fit with their values. Calabrese (2003) argues that the greater the mismatch between the new situation and the existing set of values, the greater the level of resistance.

Oreg (2006: 79–80) finds the following 'content and outcome' factors as the most significant in affecting reactions to change:

- Power and prestige – the political ramifications where individuals win or lose influential roles (authority, status) will be vigorously resisted.
- Job security – employment and income are fundamental to people's security, future life and wealth; strong survivalist factors drive resistance.

- Intrinsic rewards – autonomy and self-determination are important personal and cognitive needs. Where the new work or role is less interesting, less autonomous, less challenging, resistance increases.

Giangreco and Peccei (2005) report from their study of middle managers that reactions to change are strongly influenced by the actual content and consequences of change and, where benefits outweigh costs, reaction will be more positive and resistance lower. Assessments of impact are made regarding managing new tasks, disruption of working practice, reshaping of social relationships, and reductions in autonomy, authority and status.

Process

Hunt (1992) argues that people do not resist change per se, rather resistance is created by the way change is introduced. Similarly Paton and McCalman (2000) argue that resistance to change is more often a result of insufficient attention being paid to the process of implementing change rather than the change itself.

The 'process' view of resistance concerns how the change is proposed, information levels, management strategies and, crucially, the levels of participation and involvement.

Oreg (2006: 81–2) finds the following 'process' factors as the most significant affecting reactions to change:

- Trust in management – staff should be able to count on their managers to do what is best for them and the organization. Inspirational leaders circumvent resistance.
- Information – where this is detailed, timely, appropriate and useful, reactions to change are more positive.
- Social influence – staff are embedded within social systems forming strong attitudinal reference points. Individuals are more likely to share the reactions of their colleagues, supervisors and subordinates.

Giangreco and Peccei (2005) report that management practices such as rejecting an adversarial approach and promoting involvement of staff create more positive evaluations of the process of change. Indeed Waddell and Sohal (1998: 547) argue that one of the most critical success factors in implementing change is that managers must 'communicate and consult regularly' with their staff (see Figure 4.1) and offer the opportunity to give feedback. Perren and Megginson (1996) give an opposing view, that however morally desirable, being truthful and open may not be in the best interests of managers or organizations.

Oreg (2006) summarizes that whereas both outcomes and process factors influence how employees think (cognitive) and feel (affective) about change, their behaviour is mainly influenced by reactions to the implementation process. Imposed change faces the most resistance (O'Toole, 1995).

Understanding the context: individual, group or organizational resistance

Pardo del Val and Martinez Fuentes (2003) and Worthington (2004) argue that emergent, evolutionary change is less resisted and does not produce the same level of hostility and cynicism as imposed strategic culture change since employees feel less manipulated.

In planned approaches to change, the change is normally proposed as a 'rational' process where:

- Rational management assumes that workers will understand the change and therefore accept it.
- Resistance or non-acceptance is viewed as a psychological response to the anxiety change brings.
- Anxiety results from a failure of communication and implementation by the change agents rather than the change.
- Resistance is therefore seen as 'irrational' and resistors' objections are discounted or ignored.
- Thus a change process with minimal resistance is deemed a success.

Ford et al. (2002) suggest this takes a 'modernist' view of resistance which assumes that everyone shares the same objective reality, encounters the same change initiative and experiences it in the same context. Theories of planned change and classic management theory would therefore suggest that resistance should be quashed (Waddell and Sohal, 1998) since managers know best. Ford et al. (2002: 106) claim a 'post-modern' view sees resistance not as a 'thing' of objective reality but constructed and interpreted through social interactions and the 'reality' people create for themselves; it is therefore the nature of this reality that gives resistance its 'form, mood and flavour' and enables pluralist interpretations (Perren and Megginson, 1996).

Jarrett (2003) claims that the roots of resistance can be found in basic feelings of fear and survival operating at various levels:

- Personal defences – a denial of the reality of change.
- Group conflicts – arising from differences of perspectives.
- Organizational factors – dynamics of different interest groups perpetuate inertia.
- Institutional dynamics – history, context and environment tend to prevent innovation.

These are now explored in more detail.

Individual resistance

From an individual perspective, reasons for resistance are legion but mainly focus on the concept of loss: Buchanan and Badham (1999) report from their study of organizational politics that 81 per cent of responders agreed with the statement that one of the main sources of resistance to change comes from people defending their personal territory.

In healthcare, Worthington (2004: 62) notes resistance as stemming from loss of autonomy, erosion of traditional role boundaries and demarcation lines and the need to 'defend the symbolic realms of the organization'. Rushmer et al. (2004b) note that defensiveness fuels an unwillingness to take part in new initiatives. Similarly, Carroll and Quijada (2004: ii17) argue that 'people resist changes that undermine their hard-won expertise, status, identity, habits and understandings'.

Kegan and Lahey (2001) propose a novel solution. They claim that individuals may espouse a sincere commitment to change but unconsciously hold a psychodynamic 'competing commitment' which is entirely rational and sensible for them but works against achieving their goal. They argue that central to effective change management is uncovering this commitment so progress can be made and people can be more successful at work.

The process can be slow and painful and is based around a series of questions designed to uncover why people behave in ways that undermine their own success. These questions cover issues such as:

1 What would you like to see changed at work so you could be more effective? This usually uncovers a complaint against the organization.
2 What commitment does (your complaint) imply?
3 What are you doing (or not doing) that prevents (undermines) achieving that goal?
4 What causes discomfort or fear if you did the opposite of the undermining behaviour? In other words people imagine the actions to achieve their goal commitment and reflect on their feelings.

The final question is designed to discover the underlying 'competing commitment', their fears of achieving it and why they behave as they do:

5 By behaving like this (preventing achievement) what fearsome outcome are you determined to prevent?

The answer to this question reveals people's 'big assumptions' (Kegan and Lahey, 2001: 88) which are deeply held personal beliefs about themselves developed through lifetime relationship experiences. Using vignettes, Kegan and Lahey (2001: 87–9) demonstrate that this process is not designed to attribute blame or correct the preventing behaviour but to guide a process of understanding how these assumptions formed, surface them empathetically and provide insight in managing future behaviour:

1 A project leader's espoused commitment is open and candid communication with his subordinates. His 'preventing behaviour' was not asking his team questions about sensitive or difficult matters. This showed his 'competing commitment' was to avoid learning about things he could not fix. His 'big assumption' was that as a leader he should be able

to fix everything. If not, he would be seen as incompetent and unqualified to lead. Thus he 'prevented' himself achieving his espoused goal of open communication.

2   A manager's espoused commitment is to distribute leadership by enabling people to make decisions. Her 'preventing behaviour' was not to delegate or cascade sufficient information to enable effective decision-making. Her 'competing commitment' was having her own way, being in control, maintaining high standards and not allowing decisions she may not like. Her 'big assumption' was she thought people were not as clever as she and would make inferior decisions. Her actions therefore prevented her distributing leadership.

Kegan and Lahey (2001) argue that the process of uncovering assumptions can be painful and embarrassing but necessary to understand resistive behaviour and fully realize the opportunities of change.

Group resistance

Coghlan (1994) criticizes the literature for concentrating too much on an individual perspective. He argues that most individuals exist within some kind of work group within their organization and are bound by the social and cultural norms discussed in Chapter 7. Thus he argues, when change breaks up a team's culture and coherence and disturbs the values that hold it together, it invites resistance. He argues that evidence of group resistance comes from:

- desires to maintain team solidarity;
- rejection of outsiders;
- ensuring stability through conformity to norms;
- bonding in opposition to other groups or individuals.

This can lead to 'selective perceptions, distortions and stereotyping of other groups' (Coghlan, 1994: 20).

Entrenched attitudes related to the professional divisions of team members in healthcare can lead to conflict (see Chapter 10). These can include lack of understanding and respect for other professional roles, differences in work and learning styles and regulatory mechanisms. Oreg (2006) claims in his study of organizational restructuring that those who were surrounded by people who opposed change reported increased behavioural and affective resistance – though not a negative cognitive evaluation.

Reed (2005) notes in her study (Box 9.1) that the ward nurses exercised their resistance to change which aimed to improve patient care, passively through using their 'gatekeeping' role to control or prevent the researcher's access to the knowledge source, the patients. The effective way of exercising their limited power was to obstruct and reduce the study's potential impact.

Box 9.1

Overview

Reed (2005) reports on a study undertaken in a 'care of older people' unit in a general hospital which raises questions about the processes used to develop shared ownership in an environment unable to provide sufficient support for action research.

Background

The study developed from previous research which found that older people moving from hospital to care homes were not given adequate or appropriate opportunity to discuss their concerns with staff.

The funded study proposed to develop and implement a 'Daily Living Plan' (DLP) which aimed to specify lifestyle preferences. Completing the DLP would raise opportunities to discuss the move in more detail.

Decision and action phase 1

The study took some time to develop, with questions raised regarding scope, methods, time-scales and milestones. Six wards expressed an interest in taking part although staff were not involved in the development of the research proposal. The researcher spent much time visiting wards and meeting, discussing and gathering views about the DLP with staff. This was 'difficult and lengthy' because of time constraints and shift-work.

A project newsletter was used to facilitate project information.

In all, 37 staff from six wards and seven staff from three care homes were interviewed either individually or in focus groups regarding the design of the DLP.

Feedback phase

The draft DLP was circulated for comment. Feedback was generally positive. Researchers accepted some proposed amendments and rejected others. A final DLP was created.

Decision and action phase 2

The DLP would be actioned when patients were discharged to a care home. Nurses would raise and discuss the DLP, research ethics, consent and withdrawal with them.

Feedback phase

- Twenty-two DLPs were completed.
- Difficulties arose if patients felt pressurized into consenting and nurses felt uncomfortable asking questions.
- The researcher visited wards checking on progress and found some eligible patients had not been recruited.
- No patients were recruited in one ward despite indications that several met the criteria.

Reasons for non-recruitment were that:

- Staff were too busy, lacked time and information about the study.
- Patients were too ill or too distressed.

Attempts at deeper exploration proved fruitless.

Phase 3 fact-finding

Post-move follow-up interviews with 11 nurses who completed a DLP; 19/22 patients and 19 care home staff were recorded and transcribed.

Findings on implementing change

Positive

- DLP was seen as bridging a gap between home, hospital and care home.
- DLP was seen as broader than medical model.

Negative

- Some staff expressed negative views of care homes as routinized and impersonal.
- Care home staff were seen as less trained.
- Rigidity and routine of hospital was assumed to occur in care homes.
- DLP could raise false expectations of care homes.
- Discussing topics within the DLP could be distressing for patients.
- Only 11 nurses out of 37 completed a DLP – reasons given were 'vague and defensive' (Reed, 2005: 598).

Evaluation of resistance

Ownership

- Study did not originate from the ward nurses.
- Developed by external researchers and unit manager.
- Power differences between nurses and academics/managers/research committee.
- Status differences between academic and practical knowledge.
- No responses to the newsletter, despite requests.
- Nurses' suggestions to alter the DLP (to include medical data) were rejected as contrary to its 'patient-centred' ethos.

Sustainability

Doubts raised as to the future use of the DLP:

- Would use continue where there was little ownership and commitment?
- Funding ceased and printing further copies had cost implications.
- Use of the DLP was not Trust policy, had no budget or product champion.
- Institutional adoption would solidify the product and prevent emergent development.

(Continued)

(Continued)

Summary

Despite staff turnover, the DLP appeared to change nurses' attitudes regarding discharge of older people from hospital to care home as a major 'life-event' but particularly
the study shows the power of resistance where participants lack involvement, ownership and commitment.

Ford et al. (2002) take a different view with their post-modern perspective. They see
resistance as a socially constructed reality created through the systemic and public interactions (conversations) that people have. 'Background conversations', as symbolic language (Chapter 7) constitute an organization's culture; change attempts to shift people's
conversations but resistance resides in shared conversational patterns. This challenges
the view that resistance exists separately from the conversations that create it. Ford et al.
(2002: 109–13) propose three generic types of background 'conversations':

1 *Complacent:* This is based on historical success as proof of efficacy – 'We will succeed even
   if we remain the same'. Proposals for change are met with arguments that past strategies
   and actions have proved their worth and will continue to succeed; new goals are unnecessary; there is satisfaction with the way things are. Complacent conversations are among the
   most difficult to change since reliance on past success is the hardest obstacle to overcome
   (de Jager, 2001). Admitting that change is required is tantamount to saying that the old
   ways were wrong (Hoag et al., 2002: 12).
2 *Resigned:* This conversation is constructed around historic failure – 'This probably won't
   work either'. Self-blame predominates where people have given up trying or become half-
   hearted; they lack sufficient motivation and willingness to participate but exhibit a lack of
   belief in their ability; these beliefs justify and reinforce resistance to change.
3 *Cynical:* Similar to the 'resigned' conversation, this is built on historic failure but, rather than
   self-blame, failure is assigned to an external locus of control. The conversation is 'no one
   can make a difference – it's the way things are'. Inadequacies are located in others, the organization, the system or the world. This background, which is the bleakest, prompts attacks
   on the credibility and integrity of those proposing change or even those affiliated with
   them and will engender deep feelings of distrust.

Ford et al. (2002) argue that viewed in this way resistance is not about what is happen-
ing now but what has occurred in the past and which is assigned to the future. Therefore
standard strategies of increasing understanding and involvement will not work since
they are not at issue. What is required is to reveal the context through a 'new' conversation and begin to reframe the past through the examination of assumptions and expectations, see how these were interpreted, uncover personal responsibilities for the
outcome of dissatisfaction and develop ways to resolve tensions and differences and lay
them to rest – people must be enabled to disengage from the past.

Organizational resistance

Organizational resistance is grossly underestimated and strategies for overcoming resistance tend to misunderstand its nature, purpose and depth (Jarrett, 2003). Waddell and Sohal (1998) argue that resistance to change is built into organizations; their systems, processes, policies and procedures all contribute to inertia and constrain them to greater stability and predictability. In their exploratory study of over 500 responses by management professionals to a question about the biggest obstacles to change, Hoag et al. (2002) report that 89 per cent of responses indicated factors within the organization. Large, monopolistic health service bureaucracies do not readily incorporate change (Ashford et al., 1999) as they:

- are not usually in market-driven environments;
- have multiple goals and divergent commitments;
- are made up of a broad range of vocal constituencies with different structures and cultures;
- have limited and pre-determined funding arrangements leaving little room for re-allocation;
- are not significantly threatened by inertia;
- have difficult to devise standards and benchmarks.

Beer and Eisenstat (1996: 599), Dent and Goldberg (1999), The Royal Pharmaceutical Society (2000: 17), Hoag et al. (2002) and Pardo del Val and Martinez Fuentes (2003) all argue that obstacles to change are more likely to be in the organization's history, structure and management attitudes rather than located in individuals and include:

- Poor task co-ordination by management.
- Unclear or conflicting priorities through inadequate strategic vision.
- Inadequate organizational analysis and lack of agreement over problems (see Chapter 8).
- Top-down management style.
- Poor communication and interpersonal relations.
- Diverse lines of management and competing demands.
- Personality, status and gender factors.
- Ignorance of the social dimensions of change.

Hoag et al. (2002) report that 'management', 'organizational culture' and 'communication' emerged as the most significant obstacles to change. Oreg (2006: 93) also reports that 'trust in management' was the only variable showing significant effects on the three dimensions he studied. He summarizes that 'lack of faith in the organization's leadership was strongly related to increased reports of anger, frustration, and anxiety with respect to the change'.

Waterson (2000), reporting on a three-year study to introduce care management into a social services department (Box 9.2), uncovered resistance from staff charged with its implementation. However, her final report was 'resisted' by management, of which it was critical, through suppressing and restricting its dissemination to the very staff who had been involved in its production.

Box 9.2

Overview

Waterson (2000) discusses a study to implement 'needs-led care management' in a social services department between 1994 and 1997 where staff were expected to assess needs and purchase social care services for clients. Care management meant staff developing new skills in management, customer care, business planning, contracting and commissioning.

Senior managers set the strategy following government guidance, middle managers and social workers implemented it. Research aims were to:

- assess how workers perceived care management;
- enable participants to understand their organization and role better;
- assess progress and identify issues to be resolved.

Outcomes were three disseminated annual action research reports.

Initial exploratory and fact-finding phase

Data gathered from:

- assessors on how much care management had achieved: user empowerment, choice, needs-led assessment, tailor-made packages of care, value for money and mixed economy of care;
- policy documents, reports, operational guidelines;
- teams – over 50 staff involved;
- interviews with key senior and middle managers.

Decision and action phase 1

- Writing and dissemination of report.
- Senior management feedback.

Phase 2 fact-finding

Data gathered from providers via individual interviews with managers for specific client groups, staff groups for different services, carers' unit, user groups and voluntary sector.
Over 200 staff involved in five meetings.

Decision and action phase 2

- Writing and dissemination of report.
- Senior management feedback.

Phase 3 fact-finding

Consultative process via questionnaire to assessor and provider managers, staff and users regarding:

- The progress of care management.
- How user involvement could be promoted.
- Lessons learnt from the introduction of care management.

Two consultation meetings followed attended by 51 managers (mainly assessors); 36 completed questionnaires.

Final evaluation

- Many key staff resigned including the project originator, the task-force manager and a project worker so the project became 'inherited'.
- Constant staff changes created a lack of leadership continuity and removed a 'product champion'.
- Project aims and agenda were vague and multiple:
  - Managers: how can we meet government criteria?
  - Staff: how can we improve our service?
- Project seen as 'top-down' creating resistance and indifference from staff.
- Strength of deeply held and conflicting roles and political sensitivities were underestimated.
- Staff primarily concerned with their clients' immediate needs.
- Care management posed major threats to valued historic roles.
- Care management seen as not producing any tangible improvements to service: it promised 'individualized care packages' which could never be resourced.
- Staff were 'tired, stressed and negative' about continual change: 'it could all change tomorrow so why invest in it' (Waterson, 2000: 501).
- Many issues of implementation were seen as problems of management style rather than care management itself.
- Research exposed and challenged those in powerful positions who wanted clear 'answers' to problems.

Summary

Externally imposed change is always difficult to manage and causes powerful reactions. Staff welcomed the opportunity to have a voice and action research suited the dynamic situation.

A letter to *The Times* from a GP (Havard, 2004: 19) illustrates how positive changes to implement integrated health services are resisted and restricted by the bureaucratic systems of funding and conflicting priorities discussed above:

As a GP who is actively promoting a '1-stop shop' as part of an integrated health and social care centre, I am frustrated by the territorial nature of NHS funding. Community midwives are employed by hospital trusts not PCTs, thus the birthing unit is funded by the hospital which has no new money – the maternity unit might have to close.

The PCT could in theory fund but has historic debt.

The scheme, approved by the Department of Health exceeds the aims of the *NHS Plan* (but not the Strategic Health Authority) will provide: GP, social care (elderly, learning disability, family support), ambulance, district nursing, dental, optician, community pharmacy, podiatry, out-of-hours medical cover, birthing unit, Children's Services (health visiting, school nursing, paediatric clinics). Although we received tumultuous approval the PCT is not allowed to invest new money so we are heading for a stillbirth.

Good practice should be facilitated, not stifled.

Similarly, Fitzgerald et al. (2006) collected data from 11 case studies focusing on the roles and relationships of clinical managers across the UK acute and primary care sectors over a period of significant change (2002–05). They label one particular specialty (urological cancer services) within a recently merged three-hospital trust ('Cancer 2') as 'Resistant' to change because of a range of personal, social and organizational reasons:

- Cancer services subsumed and 'hidden' in the surgical directorate.
- Clinical director was a vascular surgeon.
- Senior urologists resigned at merger; new staff had not formed a cohesive group.
- Consultants not fully engaged with service improvements or unit management.
- Consultants did not attend either trust or cancer network meetings.
- Lack of and disputed clinical leadership in developing an improvement plan.
- 'Poor attitude' of clinicians 'obstructed' service improvement plans.

Fitzgerald et al. conclude that: 'The Cancer 2 context, however, could be regarded as more overtly *resistant* to change. Poor relationships among clinical representatives in particular ensured that service improvement initiatives were difficult to implement' (Fitzgerald et al., 2006: 78). They also note that though senior executives were aware of these problems they did not address them since their attention was diverted onto other structural changes occurring at higher levels.

Action research as a strategy for management

Coch and French (1947: 532) claim that management at the Harwood factory where they undertook their studies had long felt that 'action research is the only key to better labor-management relations'. Sixty years later Pyrch (2007: 203) considers PAR itself to be a 'form of resistance to all forms of control limiting freedom to pursue a reasoned, compassionate, committed and democratic knowledge base'. Although he argues that action research engages and empowers people, which is less likely to cause resistance, he claims that action research is itself a form of resistance against the 'unrelenting centralization and control of work' and it proposes 'democracy and devolvement of power back to the community'.

If resistance is seen as performing a useful function of continuity in its attempt to maintain equilibrium (Jarrett, 2003) and since people are more committed to changes in which they have been involved (Hedley et al. 2003) then action research provides an anti-resistant opportunity to discuss and experiment with ideas and test innovations.

Dent and Powley (2002) caution that badly applied action research methods can raise levels of resistance. This can occur when there is overuse of external consultants who may impress their own values on participants or may use organizational data uncritically, appearing as an agent of the organization. This suggests a preference for 'insider action research'. Significantly, in both action research examples where resistance is the salient feature, changes were created without the involvement of the group required to implement them.

Conclusion

Perspectives on resistance to change are themselves changing in the light of new evidence which shows resistance to be a complex, multi-dimensional concept taking many diverse forms and influenced by both personality and context as well as content and process factors which affect the way people think, feel and act towards change. Furthermore, managers who employ the assumption that no resistance equals acceptance will not engender the trust of their staff which is so vital for successful implementation, and risk fundamentally misunderstanding the change process.

Chapter summary

- Standard management literature casts reactions to change negatively as 'resistance' to be overcome.
- Individual reactions emanate from a wide range of conscious and unconscious emotions and cognitive and situational assessments.
- Reactions to change should not be immediately defined as 'resistance'.
- Resistant reactions can be rational, positive and beneficial allowing scrutiny and testing of plans and innovations.
- Overwhelmingly research indicates that where individuals perceive they will benefit from change and are involved in its implementation, resistance will be reduced.

10

Reactions to Change 2: Conflict

Introduction

Health service organizations, health professionals, managers, patient groups and patients themselves share long histories of joint working to develop constructive approaches to a wide range of healthcare issues. In most areas of health work, achieving a broad consensus on the best approach, thereby ensuring conformity, continues to be an important goal. For example, the DH voices its concerns about the number of institutions involved in developing guidelines for clinical practice:

> Guidelines should ideally be developed by consensus between primary care and secondary care groups after a systematic review of the relevant literature ... There is a risk that a plethora of local guidelines may result in conflicting recommendations which will lead to confusion and inefficient use of resources. (DH, 2004c: 1)

Similarly, in attempting to reduce costs and variations in practice where patient involvement in decision-making is concerned, the DH states:

> The existence of wide variations in referral rates, prescribing patterns and rates of use of elective surgery has underlined the extent of clinical uncertainty about the effectiveness of many common treatments and the lack of consensus in terms of appropriateness. (DH, 2003: 1)

As discussed in Chapter 4, the 'laborious consensual mechanism' (Webster, 1994: 1172) of formulating health policy (the 'cogwheel') which involved politicians working with senior doctors, nurses and administrators may have been dismantled by 'Griffiths' (Baggott, 2004) but it is clear that achieving standardized levels and quality of practice through 'one best way' agreements remains a primary concern. Lack of consensus is seen as a systemic weakness as it increases potential risk for patients, uncertainty for practitioners and potentially damaging comparisons between geographical areas, hospitals and individual practitioners.

However, meeting the demands of increased effectiveness at all levels in healthcare cannot be achieved without systematic change but this can trigger high levels of tension and conflict which have consequences on the efficiency and effectiveness of healthcare workers. As has been shown throughout this text, agreement between many factions is elusive and the organization of healthcare can be described in Morgan's term as 'a somewhat chaotic system that wishes to move in several directions at once' (1993: 215). Conflict however, is not necessarily deviant – it is a fact of life; in all organizations where there is competition for scarce resources and disputed power and control over ideas and territory, it will be present. But, since conflict is personally threatening, dealing with it is difficult since it arouses primitive emotions (Bagshaw, 1998: 206).

There are enduring views that some level of conflict is beneficial for organizations. Writing in 1925, Follett argues that:

> Conflict – difference – is here in the world, as we cannot avoid it, we should, I think use it. Instead of condemning it, we should set it to work for us … It is possible to conceive of conflict as not necessarily a wasteful outbreak of incompatibilities, but a *normal* process by which socially valuable differences register themselves for the enrichment of all concerned. (Fox and Urwick, 1973: 1–2)

Follett expresses the hope that there will always be conflict particularly the 'kind that leads to invention, to the emergence of new values' (Fox and Urwick, 1973: 7) and Jehn (1995) observes that absence of conflict is associated with organizational complacency and stagnation. Healthcare research has consistently found that many health workers avoid conflict (Skjørshammer, 2001) and nurses particularly employ a passive approach which has a detrimental effect on change outcomes (Parkin, 1999c; Valentine, 2001). If positive changes to healthcare systems and health professionals' roles occur but cause conflict, then having prior knowledge about its management will be beneficial to the leadership of teams and organizations (Choudrie, 2005).

This chapter therefore discusses:

- the relationship between change, resistance and conflict;
- the nature and meaning of conflict;
- the genesis of conflict in healthcare;
- approaches to managing conflict.

The chapter highlights two action research studies which focus on managing conflict in healthcare, one related to nursing (Taylor, 2001) and the second to midwifery (Deery, 2005), which appears to suffer from a particularly severe and significant culture of interpersonal conflict (Kirkham, 1999).

The relationship between change and conflict

The relationship between change and conflict has a long history tracing back to Machiavelli's (1532/1979: 94) celebrated sixteenth-century assertion that there is nothing 'more dangerous to handle than to introduce a new system of things for he who introduces it has all those who profit from the old system as his enemies'. Bruce and Wyman (1998) note that, at the heart of change, there are issues that generate more conflict than harmony and DiPaola and Hoy (2001) argue that conflict is the natural response to change initiatives, even from those who aim to serve clients more effectively. Following a literature review on innovation implementation, McAdam (2005) identified three key constructs:

- **Normative evaluation**: the process employees use to judge and compare an innovation against an organization's cultural norms, routines and practices developed throughout its history.
- **Legitimization**: this involves the 'sense-making' process of integrating or rejecting the innovation at the group or organization level. Innovators (who may be managers) strive for a new consensus as a model of legitimacy; employees will argue for rationality and tradition to maintain the status quo (following Machiavelli's contention above).

McAdam argues that the recursive link between normative evaluation and legitimization leads to the third construct:

- **Conflict**: this is a complex set of multi-level phenomena that is intrinsic to innovation implementation and which can be both healthy and harmful. Since employees' views of organizational values are encouraged to be normative, attempts at introducing innovation will create competition between a 'mutually incompatible set of ideas' (McAdam, 2005: 379) generating conflict at the individual, operational, group and strategic levels.

McAdam further argues that the level of conflict within a group or organization can be used as a means to assess the progress and success of innovation implementation. A potential symbiotically productive relationship between change and conflict is noted by Darling and Walker (2001: 231) who see 'that conflict can lead to change, change can lead to adaptation and adaptation can lead to survival and even prosperity'.

Resistance or conflict

Resistance and conflict are often linked and used synonymously with little attempt to draw out differences, but, reviewing the research and theoretical literature reveals clear distinctions between the two concepts. Chapter 9 argues that the nature and cause of resistance is located within the organizational or individual's work system where there are forces which maintain the status quo. Its management is focused on the means of 'overcoming' it through strategies of involvement, re-contextualization or explanation. The origins of resistance tend to be organizational whereas conflict is emotional and originates within people.

Whereas 'resistance' was defined as 'making a stand against' and speaks of a reluctance to become engaged or a systemic drag on involvement, 'conflict' comes from the Latin 'confligere' meaning 'to strike together', to 'clash' or 'fight'. This has a more aggressive, hostile even violent tone focused on deeper and more contentious differences of opinion.

Where resistance is 'overcome' (and its antonym is 'surrender') conflict tends to be 'resolved' through a negotiation and bargaining process to reach its antonym of 'agreement'. Whereas worker 'participation' is the strategy of choice for overcoming resistance it has little impact in dealing with differences.

The nature and meaning of conflict

Anderson (2005) argues that the potential for conflict is almost limitless occurring on any scale from the personal level within the mind of one person, spilling out into the community involving groups and extending to outright warfare between nation states. He claims that individual conflict may be the simplest stage but that inter or intra-group conflict is much more likely. Follett (Fox and Urwick, 1973: 1) argues that conflict should not be thought of as 'warfare' but simply as 'the appearance of difference, difference of opinions, of interests'. Rahim (1985: 81–2) describes conflict as 'an "interactive state" manifested in disagreement, differences, or incompatibility, within or between individuals and groups'. He classifies organizational conflict as 'intrapersonal, interpersonal, intra-group and inter-group'. Jehn (1995) defines conflict as perceptions by parties that they hold discrepant views or have interpersonal incompatibilities; conflict behaviours are the consequences of the perceived discrepancies although conflict can be present without physical manifestations.

DiPaola and Hoy state that: 'Conflict begins when an individual or group feels negatively affected by another person or group. It may occur in interpersonal encounters between two colleagues, in decision-making teams, between work groups, or in board meetings' (DiPaola and Hoy, 2001: 238). They further argue that the larger and more diverse the group, the greater the potential for conflict, because greater diversity amongst group members results in wider differences in goals, perceptions, preferences and beliefs. In healthcare, with its multitude of groups, conflict is particularly likely to occur at the boundaries or interfaces where different occupational groups strive for control over scarce or limited resources or over disputed territorial ownership (Drife and Johnson, 1995). However this can provide positive opportunities for collaborative work, role change and learning and the potential to develop alternative means of enhancing standards and services.

Causes of conflict

At the superficial level, there is general consensus over the causes of conflict. Donaldson (1995) argues that conflict will exist wherever individual or group interests diverge and when values or goals are at odds with those of the external environment. Anderson (2005: 244–5) subsumes the causes of conflict under three headings:

- The central issue.
- The people involved (either as individuals or groups).
- The organization and structure where conflict occurs.

He suggests that the most important causes 'relate to the characteristics of the groups involved, their interests, values, and aims' (2005: 245).

Zartman (1991: 12) however takes a different view. He classifies conflict in the following ways:

1 A simple contest of opposing parties (interpersonal or inter-group) each attempting to impose a unilateral solution to a problem. The more powerful party is likely to prevail. Here resolution focuses on a negotiated multilateral formula acceptable to both parties. This is the common view of conflict. Where parties refuse to work collaboratively, conflict is likely to increase.
2 Conflict is intrapersonal or intra-group and occurs when the cost–benefit ratio of actions and decisions do not meet acceptable levels in the context.
3 Conflict is more complex and is related to changes in systems and regimes: accepted patterns of working are challenged, become strained, break down and a new order has to be identified and established through a long, uncertain and evolutionary process.

In healthcare, Skjørshammer (2001) notes that the main reason for feuds in hospitals is the conflict over the co-ordination of care required to improve quality and reduce costs whereas Drife and Johnson (1995) claim that it is usually triggered by disputes over territory and the inappropriate use of power as illustrated in Box 10.1.

Box 10.1

Overview

Taylor (2001) reports on a study with 12 experienced nurses meeting with a facilitator for one hour per week for 16 weeks. The meetings were designed to facilitate reflective practice in order to raise awareness of practice problems, work through problem-solving processes systematically to uncover constraints against effective nursing practice and improve the quality of care. The group identified dysfunctional nurse–nurse relationships to work on and transform through the application of action research methods.

Literature indicates that nurses undergo socialization into female roles of 'care-giving'.

Demands can create a sense of powerlessness which can turn into negative behaviour towards colleagues which is then maintained through strategies of denial, minimization and ritualization.

Initial exploratory cycle – weeks 1–3

The development of the group:

- Packages detailing reflective practice, action research methods, articles and journals were given to participants.
- Introductions and rules emphasized dynamics of trust, openness, privacy, confidentiality, respect for others and active listening.
- Participants required to refrain from criticism, advice and 'fixing'.
- Disclosures only made if comfortable but climate ensured all had a 'voice'.
- Participants encouraged to share ideas raised from reflective practice.

Second cycle – weeks 4–7

Sharing issues from practice:

- Example 1 focused on advocacy, speaking up where difficulty was perceived in doctor–nurse relations and professional role expectations.
- Example 2 raised issues of victimization which led to discussions of betrayal by peers, fear of powerful figures, clinical incompetence, and the need for 'fearful obedience'. Issues were grouped under two main areas:
- Professional relationships:

  - Doctor–nurse, patient–nurse and nurse–nurse relationships.
  - Gender, hierarchy, communication and peer pressure in decision-making.
  - Power, advocacy and recognition as professionals.

- Professional identity:

  - Guilt and regret 'I have not performed well'.
  - Lack of confidence and self-esteem, blaming not learning from the past.
  - Requirements to be 'invincible and perfect', and 'accountable and achieve'.

Plans made to focus on and address issues in professional relationships.

Third cycle – weeks 8–16

Group expressed progress and appreciation of the open dynamics of reflection and sharing but also cautioned that participants should engage in research rather than a 'witch-hunt' of unfavoured individuals and should ensure anonymity and confidentiality.

Aimed to develop an action plan to deal with dysfunctional nurse–nurse relationships (bullying, betrayal, professional jealousy, misuse of power) through consideration of commonalities and principles of examples discussed:

- Determinants of conflict:

  - History of nursing.
  - Cultural norms in roles and relationships.
  - Political aspects of interpersonal communication.
  - Low self-esteem in originator.
  - Gender issues.

Strategies resolving conflicts

Designed to empower the group to act effectively beyond organizational constraints and focus on a 'problem-solving' approach:

- Develop a culture of positive strokes and acknowledgements.
- Empower nurses themselves to develop appropriate policies.
- Deal with originator directly using policies and procedures (cognitive).
- Act through strong leadership.

(Continued)

(Continued)

- Examine and target action on underlying situational determinants.
- Encourage mutual nurse–nurse support.
- Use evidence and document procedures.
- Use line management appropriately.
- Build conflict management skills or request facilitator's assistance.
- Present a 'united front' to line management.

Strategies should be enacted through:

- Face-to-face meetings.
- Moderate and supportive attitudes.
- Reflective listening and paraphrasing.
- Awareness of difference between assertion and aggression.
- Maintaining confidentiality.

Evaluation

Participant stories and journal entries showed mixed outcomes. Effective communication required courage and clarity of purpose. Self management and control was essential.

Summary

There are no quick fixes to complex deep-seated emotional situations. Difficult healthcare situations often prevent clear, open communication and can militate against mutual respect and co-operation. Collaborative work should continue to effect cultural change in nursing relationships.

Conflict as positive or negative

Historically, conflict has been characterized as negative since it creates tensions between individuals and teams in their personal and professional relationships and can reduce effectiveness as it diverts attention from the task (Medina et al., 2005). Juhl et al. (2004) and Medina et al. (2005) argue that the traditional view of conflict, still endorsed by today's managers and employees, is that it is destructive and should be eliminated, avoided or resolved as soon as possible. Morgan (1993: 214) argues that 'unitary managers' expect their staff to obey and respect the right of managers to manage hence conflict is seen as an unwanted and unnecessary intrusion. However, within an interactionist philosophy a certain level of conflict is considered to be valuable for an organization and should be encouraged to enhance both team and organizational performance. Morgan (1993: 215) suggests that the hallmark of 'pluralist managers' is that they accept the inevitability of organizational politics and see that conflict can benefit the organization and can be used as a means to achieve desired ends. The interactionist approach, concerning social dynamics of interpreting meanings and perceptions, suggests that managers should attempt to resolve conflicts that hinder the orga-nization but actively stimulate conflict intensity to a degree that maintains the organization as an innovative and responsive unit. Similarly Follett (Fox and Urwick, 1973), through defining conflict as 'difference' or 'diversity', claims it would be wrong to eliminate it since diversity is an essential feature of life and should not be feared. Anderson (2005) argues that conflict can be positive where channels of communication are open and solutions can be found through collaboration and negotiation but where coercion and dominance are used or conflict is left unresolved, it is destructive. Mike Brearley (2000: 1141), the ex-England cricket captain and a psychoanalyst argues that creativity requires conflicting ideas; para-phrasing William Blake, he asserts, that 'without contrariety [*sic*] there is no progression'[1] and notes that conflict and tensions appear in all successful teams.

Indeed, the opportunity for argument, debate and dissent is at the very heart of the democratic process. Evidence suggests that conflict is beneficial to team performance and suppressing it may reduce creativity, innovation, performance, quality of decisions, and communication between group members (De Dreu, 1997; Medina et al., 2005). Mill also observes (1910: 247) 'in all human affairs conflicting influences are required to keep one another alive and efficient'.

Morgan (1993: 216) and Parkin (1999c: 278) summarize that conflict can:

- counter tendencies towards lethargy and promote reflection;
- suppress groupthink;
- create an atmosphere where it is risky to take things for granted;
- encourage evaluation which challenges conventional wisdom and increases the quality of decisions;
- encourage groups to search for new solutions to underlying problems through cost–benefit analyses;
- facilitate mutual accommodation through exploration and negotiation;
- be essential to realize the benefits of collaboration.

Although Morgan argues for the need for conflict and for managers to judge and main-tain an optimum level, he does not discriminate between different types of conflict which is now considered an important part of the equation.

Functional and dysfunctional conflict

Although terminology varies (see Table 10.1), many writers make a distinction between conflict that is functional (beneficial) or dysfunctional (Jehn, 1995) which have differ-ent consequences. Parkin (1999c) claims that although the distinction can be a difficult judgement, it is the key to understanding 'productive' conflict.

In relation to change, McAdam (2005) argues simply that 'constructive' conflict encourages innovation implementation whereas 'destructive' conflict discourages it.

---

1 'Without contraries is no progression. Attraction and Repulsion, Reason and Energy, Love and Hate, are necessary to Human existence', William Blake (1794), Plate 3, *The Marriage of Heaven and Hell*. Jura, France: Trianon Press.

Table 10.1 Alternative terminology for functional and dysfunctional conflict

Functional	Dysfunctional
Cognitive	Affective
Task	Relationship
Productive	Unproductive
Constructive	Destructive
Substantive	Emotional
Healthful	Relational
Liberating	

Sources: Jehn (1995); De Dreu (1997); Passos and Caetano (2005).

Other theorists widen the definition. Functional conflict focuses on disagreements which are rooted within the content and issues of the task, the surrounding decisions, opinions, ideas and points of view. It is more intellectual in origin and relates to the relative importance of the task, decisions taken, resources, policies, procedures and roles (Jehn, 1995; Parkin, 1999c; Passos and Caetano, 2005).

Functional conflict is seen as positively enhancing group performance as it:

- increases understanding of alternative and multiple views;
- stimulates questioning and effective use of information;
- improves the evaluation of alternatives;
- enhances critical thinking and decision-making processes.

Anderson (2005) notes that conflict has a tendency to grow from an awareness that differences exist to a hardening of attitudes through to open hostility. This latter stage is dysfunctional and is mainly based on strong emotional, personal and relational components. Dysfunctional conflict is rooted in animosity, hostility, intolerance and incompatibility between people and can contain affective states of hatred and jealousy (DiPaola and Hoy, 2001; Medina et al., 2005). Disagreements can become 'personalized' with friction, frustration and personality clashes over personal norms and taste (Jehn, 1995; Parkin, 1999c; Medina et al., 2005) and is the type of conflict illustrated in Box 10.2.

Box 10.2

Overview

Deery (2005) reports on the first study of its kind in midwifery with eight NHS community midwives exploring their views and experiences of support and supervision in practice through three phases of action research using interviews and focus groups. Midwifery has struggled with the pace and nature of long-term, large-scale change leading to recruitment and retention problems compounded by a culture of support

---

given to mothers in stark contrast to impoverished intra-group and management support, leading to serious occupational 'burnout'.

Phase one

Preparatory work included meeting managers, preparing midwives on the nature of the study, gaining consent, and agreeing on disclosure and confidentiality.

In-depth, pre-piloted, taped, transcribed and anonymized individual interviews carried out. Areas of enquiry included:

- Life as a community midwife.
- Attitudes towards work.
- Levels of support provided for midwives.
- Change areas identified.

Findings

Each transcript read four or five times:

- The full extent of midwives' stress and lack of support became apparent.
- Organizational structures were insensitive to their professional and personal needs.
- Their working relationships were 'unsupported, constraining and intimidating' (Deery, 2005: 170).
- Their 'voices' were silenced or rejected.
- 'Emotion work' by midwives is not acknowledged or understood by midwives themselves, their managers or the organization.
- Government policies threatened midwives' ways of working and well-being.
- Change seen as 'extra work'. They were overwhelmed with demands and workload.
- 'Team-midwifery' seen as an imposition.
- Complaints about underlying nastiness, dreadful dynamics and personality differences leading to arguments and 'bickering'.
- An image of 'pseudo-cohesion' was projected as a defence mechanism.
- Work-related issues dealt with superficially, manipulatively or destructively to sabotage intentions.
- Denial and avoidance strategies used with interpersonal issues.
- Data indicated they were 'overwhelmed' by their interpersonal relationships.

Midwives were offered but were reluctant to engage in data analysis seeing it as 'extra work'.

Phase two

Two focus groups:

1. To reflect on interviews and devise a plan to create a collaborative and mutual support mechanism.
2. To construct the practice-based support mechanism (CS).

(Continued)

(Continued)

First focus group: findings

Plans to facilitate a non-hierarchical participatory approach were not realized as some midwives dominated and some were muted. This replicated the team's normal functioning where sensitive interpersonal conflict and confrontation dominated.

- Support needs were not being met.
- Lack of consistent management.
- The participation and collaboration required in action research was found to be unfamiliar to the group.
- Exposed a culture of fear and isolation.

It was felt that clinical supervision (CS) may help.

First focus group: action

A mental health professional agreed to facilitate two workshops on the nature and benefits of CS and midwives' roles.
   A third was offered but refused by the group despite an identified need.

Second focus group: findings

Midwives interacted angrily with the researcher and showed signs of reluctance to continue, frustration and lack of support.
   Researcher contacted senior managers to negotiate extra cover, support and funding.

Second focus group: action

Midwives identified a potential supervisor and planned, through contracts, to attend CS fortnightly for 6 months. In reality attendance was poor as 'they had no time in which to undertake CS' and contracts were broken.

Phase three

Individual interviews with five remaining midwives to include:

- Nature, expectations, actions taken and outcomes of CS.
- Relevance of CS to midwifery.
- Changes in practice caused by CS.

Findings

- The challenges of the project seemed too much for the midwives to manage.
- Regarding CS: beneficial, necessary but an extra chore with no time to devote to it.
- Did not keep to CS ground-rules.
- Dealing with dysfunctional dynamics was difficult to address.
- Rather than use CS constructively, poor attitudes and work patterns persisted.

Evaluation

Midwives spent their working life in cultural conflict: meeting the needs of others but not meeting their own needs nor taking the opportunity provided to address the deficit. Midwives work in a bureaucratic hierarchical system intolerant of different ways of thinking. They were not prepared educationally for group functioning and ill-prepared for collaborative work which provided the means to promote intra-group support.

Summary

Action research was found to be highly appropriate to research rapidly changing maternity settings as it accommodates the unpredictability, complex and messy nature of dynamic clinical practice situations through collaboration, democracy and empowerment.

Dysfunctional conflict has a negative effect on group performance and satisfaction as well as psychological well-being (Medina et al., 2005) as it:

- limits information processing;
- saps energy and focus away from the task;
- reduces decision-making effectiveness and commitment to the decision.

Although Passos and Caetano (2005) find no relationship between conflict and either team performance or satisfaction in their study, they suggest that national culture may affect the way individuals and groups interpret conflict.

Jehn (1995) cautions, however, that high levels of task or cognitive conflict can spill over into affective conflict and become detrimental to productive work, especially if it is not resolved; the benefits of task conflict may disappear if affective conflict increases (Medina et al., 2005). Jehn further analysed that where groups performed routine tasks, conflict over content (cognitive) was detrimental since members perceived it as unimportant and continued in their routine ways. She reports that cognitive conflict is only beneficial in non-routine situations which prompt open discussion and critical evaluation of material. Affective conflict tends to be detrimental regardless of the type of task performed.

Managing conflict

Rahim (1985: 82) argues that since a moderate amount of conflict is necessary to achieve organizational effectiveness, it is more instructive to act in terms of conflict 'management' rather than 'resolution' since this does not advocate its elimination. McElhaney (1996) refers to a study which found that American managers rated 'conflict

Table 10.2   Theoretical approaches to conflict management

Blake and Mouton (1964)	Thomas and Kilmann (1974)	Rahim and Bonoma (1979)	Follett (Fox and Urwick, 1973)
Forcing	Competing	Dominating	Domination
Withdrawing	Avoiding	Avoiding	
Smoothing	Accommodating	Obliging	
Sharing	Compromising	Compromising	Compromise
Problem-solving	Collaborating	Integrating	Integration

management' equal or higher in importance to the management tasks of planning, communication or decision-making. What is required is the ability to guide conflict into its most creative mode so that its benefits are gained to achieve a win–win outcome for the contesting parties while avoiding any destructive costs (Bruce and Wyman, 1998; Passos and Caetano, 2005).

Medina, et al. (2005: 228) lay down some fundamental principles for managers to improve conflict management:

- Understand the type and intensity of conflict taking place.
- Encourage open discussion of task related issues.
- Mitigate or resolve 'relationship' conflicts as soon as possible.
- Attend to the level of conflict because of its interactive effects.

One of the first theorists to write about conflict, Follett (Fox and Urwick, 1973) claims that there are three main ways of 'dealing' with it though other writers have devised five (Table 10.2).

Domination or *competition*: this is a power-oriented mode with the victory of one side, through use of authority or threats, over the other. This is, Follett claims, the easiest and quickest and used by higher management (Rahim, 1985), but is an impediment to progress and the least successful in the long term.

Compromise: here each side yields something in order to gain peace and enable actions to continue. Compromise is the most common and accepted approach as it is the way most people settle controversies through yielding and gaining concessions and is the basis of unionized collective bargaining, yet Follett also argues that if compromise is used exclusively, it does not deal with the fundamentals which will continue to return. Furthermore, it only deals with what exists and produces nothing new.

Avoidance: although not in Follett's vocabulary, it is applied significantly in healthcare. Avoidance involves withdrawing from conflict situations, not acknowledging its presence and declining to confront or address it. This delays dealing with pressing issues or leaves them unresolved which affects the achievement of goals. This style is unproductive and leads to negative results for the team and organization (Parkin, 1999c). DiPaola and Hoy (2001) claim that children are taught not to disagree and that in many cultures arguing is discouraged. This, they propose, creates a culture where adults are unaccustomed to confronting uncomfortable conflict situations which are avoided.

Accommodating: this signifies attempts by parties to satisfy the concerns of others while neglecting their own. It is the opposite of competing and contains aspects of self-sacrifice.

Finally, Follett (Fox and Urwick, 1973: 9) describes *integration* (alternatively termed *problem-solving* (see Chapter 8) or *collaborating* (see Figure 4.1 and Table 10.2)), as a far more profitable and mature way of managing conflict where differences are brought into the open; the conflict is uncovered where it can be examined since 'evaluation often leads to a revaluation'. It involves openness, information exchange and examination of differences (Rahim, 1985) which frames conflict as a mutual learning opportunity, the creation of something new and the development of an organizational memory (DiPaola and Hoy, 2001). The focus should remain on the issue rather than the person.

Kakabadse (2000: 12) too asserts that it is important to create an environment where 'the pronouncing of views, the asking of questions, the entering into deep debate and emerging with a declaring of intent' is a vital process in which to engage to enable a move towards a more cohesive team suitable for organizational leadership. Where team members believe they are in a co-operative situation, where they can express their opinions and where mutually beneficial goals are primary rather than in a competitive situation in which they are trying to outdo each other, conflict will be viewed as constructive and work will be enhanced. Rahim (1985) states that this is the most effective strategy since openness will ensure that the skills and information will be shared by the parties to formulate successful solutions and implementation.

Behavioural styles

Darling and Walker (2001: 232–35) extend these well rehearsed approaches by adding a 'behavioural' dimension. They discuss four 'behavioral styles' and their conflict management orientations which indicate how individuals work and interact with others in conflict management situations:

- People-oriented 'relaters' reflect high emotional responsiveness and low assertiveness. They are sensitive towards others and their needs and use empathy and understanding. Relaters prefer stability, are likeable, easy-going, co-operative and slow to change.

  - Relaters are generally uncomfortable with conflict situations.

- Process-oriented 'analysers' are precise, logical and systematic, gathering and evaluating evidence before acting and are objective and well organized. They have lower levels of emotional responsiveness and assertiveness and are industrious and objective. They tend to resist compromise in conflict situations.

  - Analysers tend to be uncomfortable with change hence can contribute to organizational conflict.

- Action-oriented 'directors' have lower levels of emotional responsiveness but higher levels of assertiveness. They are task-oriented 'doers' focusing on results, they are confident, competitive, independent, decisive and determined.

  - Directors can be challenging and take a lead in conflict management.

- Creative orientated 'socializers' integrate high levels of emotional responsiveness and assertiveness, are innovative risk-takers and persuasive but are friendly, enthusiastic and outgoing.

  - Socializers' creativity can make people uncomfortable and contribute to conflict.

Darling and Walker (2001) recognize that these interactive styles can contribute to organizational conflict but claim that understanding the styles and attempting to incorporate aspects of other styles (such as assertiveness or responsiveness) can be the key to more effective interaction in conflict situations.

Conflict in healthcare

Skjørshammer (2001) notes the paucity of empirical studies examining conflict management between professionals but his Norwegian hospital-based study uncovers some valuable insights. Unusually his data differentiate between conflict perspectives and management styles of doctors and nurses. Skjørshammer (2001) discovers that, out of the range of management styles available and regardless of professional background, department or hierarchical level, health professionals tend to use only three styles, avoidance, forcing and negotiation (compromise) (see Table 10.2), but that 'avoidance' was the most common strategy of choice. Particularly he found that doctors have a higher threshold for conflict than other staff since their professional self-concept and culture enables them to tolerate higher levels of stress. In many cases however 'avoidance' was functional since it is a strategy that recognizes the 'pre-existing patterns of resolution which define the direction and relative power of interdependence between involved parties' (Skjørshammer, 2001: 15). This refers to the perceived importance of doctors' tasks and definitional power in controlling resources including knowledge and skills and meeting the aims of healthcare thereby gaining 'the upper hand'; a view endorsed by Drife and Johnson (1995) who argue that the dominant healthcare culture (see Table 7.1) is clinical because of its powerful networks and high public credibility.

In the UK, Salvage and Smith (2000: 1019) note that relationships between doctors and nurses have never been straightforward; there are differences of power, perspective, education, status, class, and gender which, as Chapter 7 indicates, lead to 'tribal warfare as often as peaceful coexistence'. They continue:

> Nurses are becoming more assertive, educated and competent than ever before … Doctors, puzzled and unaccustomed to being challenged, are themselves resentful at the apparent undervaluing of their competence, knowledge, and skill by nurses, the public, and policymakers. Everyone is confused. (Salvage and Smith, 2000: 1019)

Chuang et al. (2004) claim that evidence shows that greater diversity of status, age, gender, race and ethnicity within and between groups generates negative effects and a decrease in performance. Alternatively, groups who share values interpret problems and events similarly, are less likely to fall out over goals, tasks and actions and will show tolerance and respect.

Davies (2000) differs in arguing that inter-group collaboration, especially between doctors and nurses, is successful because of the groups' differences; group diversity can achieve much more than like-minded groups but this diversity has to be acknowledged and valued by all sides.

Nurses appear to overuse 'avoidance' and under-use 'collaboration' (Valentine, 2001) as do midwives (Kirkham, 1999). Valentine argues that nurses may avoid conflict because of their orientation to caring for others and a sense of powerlessness in relation to other healthcare workers. High avoiders cause co-ordination problems and delay decisions and need training and support in participatory methods (Fagan, 1985). Mullally (2003), England's Chief Nursing Officer argues that in nursing 'niceness', the backing off in challenging situations, is a tyranny that avoids conflict and one which the profession has yet to lose. Under-using collaboration highlights that differences of opinions are not being used as learning opportunities or to solve problems and nursing issues are not being dealt with adequately (Fagan, 1985).

Conclusion

Similarly to resistance, conflict is a real event in change management but should not habitually be seen as having negative effects. Where conflict can be maintained as 'cognitive' and the management strategy is integrative or problem-solving, constructive change is more likely to occur. Alternatively, where conflict is affective in nature and the management strategy is forcing or coercive, change will be inhibited.

Chapter summary

- Conflict is a common response to change but should be distinguished from 'resistance'.
- Theorists have distinguished between:
  - Cognitive conflict which focuses on the task and can be functional in promoting team performance.
  - Emotional conflict, which focuses on interpersonal and 'personalized' differences and can be dysfunctional, reducing team effectiveness.
- There is a range of strategies used to manage conflict. In healthcare, evidence overwhelmingly indicates that 'avoidance' is preferred.
- A 'problem-solving' collaborative approach is more successful in maintaining 'cognitive' conflict leading to higher quality decisions and more successful change.

11

Strategies for Implementing Change

Introduction

Leading, managing and implementing change successfully, whether at individual, team, department or organization levels, is often seen as the pinnacle of achievement in professional and managerial practice. It is simultaneously difficult, exciting, fearful, taxing and satisfying but does not occur through chance, routine or drift. At the most basic level it should be thought through and co-ordinated, but any idea of innovation in a complex organization presents an immense challenge. To complicate matters, none of the highly developed 'rational' models of change that dominate the management literature reflect the real world or can prepare practitioners for the implementation stage, but, sooner or later actions have to be taken.

This chapter aims to bring together many of the major theoretical aspects from previous chapters and reinterpret them as a range of practical implementation strategies which are available, to a greater or lesser extent, to frontline practitioners. It draws together key concepts from Figures 4.1, 6.4 and 8.1 and, with further discussion, provides a compendium of responses for those wishing or planning to implement change in healthcare and manage any ensuing resistance and conflict. The compendium, seen as a reservoir of strategic actions, is not nor can be exhaustive since each situation, organization and team profile will differ.

Hunt sets out the challenges and difficulties of implementing change:

> For any manager, change is a muddling through, energy draining activity characterized by stop-go tactics. It involves selling information, motivating resistors and hoping that some dominant logic will encourage actors to internalize the change and thereby change their behaviours. Unfortunately, there is no adequate theory which explains the social, psychological, managerial or structural processes of change in organizations. (Hunt, 1992: 260)

Beer and Eisenstat (1996: 598) note that there is a gap between intervention theory and practice because a research base for developing organizations does not exist. They argue that implementation must focus on 'strategy and organization, structure and behaviour, analysis and emotion, internal organizational arrangements and the context in which the organization operates'. In healthcare particularly, these are complex and challenging demands.

Eccles (1994: 63) is clear about what implementation means: 'Implementation is action. It is not planning or thinking about action, nor persuading others or making decisions … It is the action itself … with all its attendant elements of error, frustration, turmoil, expense and confusion'. It is also the 'central hub' of action research (Bridges and Meyer, 2007: 391). Actions, however, cannot occur in isolation from the context and have to be underpinned and influenced by the 'interpersonal processes' of 'communication', 'consultation', 'collaboration' and 'co-ordination' shown in Figure 4.1.

Gill (2006) notes that the term strategy derives from the Greek '*strategos*' originally referring to a General in command of an army but over time its meaning has widened to be seen as a 'journey plan' or 'route map' (2006: 178), involving the creation, by senior management or governments, of long-term plans and competitive positioning. Though familiar in healthcare this is now seen as outmoded where a 'top-down vision and direction should be replaced by bottom-up initiatives from people who are closest to the customer' (Gill, 2006: 197). Potter et al. (1994) argue that national strategies may be important for setting a direction and framework but have little effect on operational staff in the field; by the time they reach department and team level, they have lost all impact. The role for senior management now is to clearly define and frame the vision and mission and 'empower people to pursue them' (Gill, 2006: 180).

This chapter therefore considers:

- Fundamental principles for implementing change based on the philosophy of action research.
- The content, nature and substance of change.
- Influences on strategy choice.
- A restatement of core concepts as strategies including:
  - culture and structure;
  - leadership;
  - communication;
  - participation;
  - team learning.

The role of action research in strategy implementation

In their seminal and often quoted discussion on strategies for effecting change in human systems, Chin and Benne (1976: 32) single out the 'normative-re-educative' strategy as one focusing on individuals as active learners who do not passively wait for and respond to stimuli but consciously work towards shaping a better fit between organizational relations and environmental demands and resources. They emphasize the significance of Lewin's vision of the interrelationship between research, education and action as contributing to this strategy particularly through:

- identifying need for change;
- developing collaborative relationships;
- solving human problems;
- working through improved knowledge and patterns of action in meeting those needs.

They argue (Chin and Benne, 1976: 32) that 'these convictions led Lewin to emphasize action research as a strategy of changing, and participation in groups as a medium for re-education' which is in contrast and preference to the 'power-coercive' strategy they also discussed. These arguments remain today: Bridges and Meyer (2007) note the close relationship between action research and successful strategies for implementing change particularly its emphasis on democracy and participation; Elsey and Lathlean (2006) argue that action research provides the ideal forum for bringing together different levels of staff with service users; and Burgess-Macey and Rose (1997: 61) endorse action research as the 'ultimate in ownership'. Galvin et al.'s (1999) study in Box 11.1 illustrates the opportunities for role and skill development in a multi-disciplinary healthcare team, and the painful 'disconfirmation' process in new learning and team growth through crossing boundaries. The study also develops theory in terms of a new model which would not have occurred if this had been an imposed management strategy.

Box 11.1

Overview

Galvin et al. (1999) report on complex changes made within a large five GP, 7,700 patient surgery to develop better team working, professional roles and partnerships.

A large number of practice nurses had been employed eroding the roles of other staff, especially health visitors who felt threatened and undervalued. GPs felt frustrated over demands on their time and other limitations such as hierarchical relationships, inter-professional disputes, skill mix and inappropriate use of team skills.

Aims: to gain user perspectives about the service, examine nursing work and roles, clarify core and specialist skills, identify areas for change and define new roles through developing a new model of team working.

Exploratory and planning phase

Data were collected from multiple sources:

- Patient focus group interviews: examining access, opportunities for service development and patient involvement.
- Interviews with a GP, practice manager and community nursing area manager.
- User satisfaction survey – surgery and consultations.
- Task analysis: recording a typical working week and identifying professional practice boundaries.

- Team workshops: examining data and proposing changes and new roles.
- Reflective diaries: project and nursing teams consider views on group dynamics and the process of action research.

Decision and action phase

Patients felt that the team was efficient and caring with high levels of satisfaction but had concerns over continuity of care, location of services, child health, clinic times and aspects of wound care.

The GP, practice manager and area manager felt services were formed around the teams' interests and expertise and the professionals' view of patients' needs. Knowledge needed to be shared in order to provide a holistic service.

The nursing team was keen to develop practice services in relation to:

- working across professional boundaries;
- identifying core and professionally specific skills;
- responding to user feedback;
- identifying organizational change.

Areas considered for change to achieve a patient-led service:

- A multi-skilled nurse practitioner working in both surgery and community.
- Proposals for:
  - health promotion;
  - social benefit advice;
  - pre-operative assessment;
  - asthma and diabetes management;
  - record keeping;
  - clearer leadership for the nursing team and support workers.

Agreed areas for change included:
  - child health;
  - leg ulcer management;
  - cardio-vascular health.

All practice team members were involved in decisions and organization of new services.

Second phase

- Meetings held to support staff in the new ventures.
- Each new service proceeded at different rates.
- Time constraints and busy schedules caused some breakdown in communications and increased intra-team tensions.
- Strong opinions were expressed about the 'new ways of working'.
- Different roles were worked out and agreed.

(Continued)

(Continued)

The leg ulcer clinic opening was delayed adding to conflicts. A new protocol and assessment tool was prepared, though at the initial clinic nurses felt they lacked full understanding, causing further tensions.

In cardio-vascular health a new assessment tool and patient information sheet was adopted.

A new model of team working was produced where traditional role boundaries could be crossed providing opportunity for flexibility and outreach work. Three new roles were needed: a team facilitator, a primary healthcare nurse and a generic support worker.

Summary

The project created some difficulties and successes. Collaboration was achieved though considerable effort was required around areas of communication, understanding roles and competing demands. Group boundaries and roles became confused as would be expected when introducing boundary flexibility. It was not feasible to rush action research as time was needed to acclimatize to new systems. Locating leadership was difficult.

Ongoing phases

- Further moves away from rigid role demarcation.
- Piloting of new model.

Statement of fundamental principles for implementation

Implementation strategies are underpinned by research which has consistently indicated that there are enduring leitmotifs to the successful management of change. These include:

1 Creating the climate for innovation: Chapter 1 rehearses Plsek and Wilson's (2001) claim that this can be achieved through focusing on four key areas – direction pointing; managing boundaries; gaining permission; and managing resources.
2 Every organization, team context and culture is unique and influenced by the variables set out in Chapter 4 and the features identified from fact-finding processes in Chapter 8. What works in one context will not necessarily work in another.
3 Methods of implementing change are infinite and it is unrealistic to try to code them as discrete as they invariably overlap (Hunt, 1992). Since organizations are a complex mix of forces there is a need for a multifaceted strategy to influence embedded behaviours (Hendry, 1996).
4 Hunt's position that there is no adequate theory available to explain the processes of change indicates that both practitioners and strategies must be flexible according to developing circumstances. There is no recipe which ensures success and relying on a single fixed strategy is unwise.

5 Therefore, implementation strategies, especially in large healthcare organizations, cannot be 'straightforward or linear' and should 'contain an important element of emergent and unplanned activity' (Elsey and Lathlean, 2006: 172). Martins and Terblanche (2003: 70) stress that the values of 'flexibility over rigidity' and 'freedom over control' are core values in innovation.

6 Strategies should be open, democratic, involving and promote learning. Evidence has consistently shown that participation builds ownership which reduces opposition. Employee participation in fact-finding, analysis, problem-identification and solving, development of responses and evaluation of results, translates into ongoing collaborative actions (Bruce and Wyman, 1998).

The content, nature or substance of change

Potential change initiatives are outlined in Table 1.1.

Eccles (1994:13) claims that strategy implementation will nearly always involve:

- revising policies for the organization and group;
- developing new individual/group performance criteria;
- modifying structure, systems and behaviour;
- developing and learning new skills; unlearning old skills.

The action research studies in Boxes 11.1 and 11.2 illustrate each of Eccles' points.

Davies et al. (2000) note that wholesale and simultaneous change on all aspects of organizational culture is unfeasible and undesirable. They claim that successful starts need to take into account the needs, fears, and motivations of staff at all levels. As Huczynski and Buchanan (2001) argue, the human aspects of change have to be managed as carefully as the technical, organizational and structural aspects.

Influences on strategy choice

Eccles (1994: 11) argues that formulation of strategy is required when:

- A new vision or goal is produced.
- A new way of pursuing the vision or goal is created.
- A reorganization is undertaken.
- The conditions for survival radically alter requiring a change in approach, objectives and behaviour.

Furthermore the magnitude of change will determine the choice of strategy; levels of magnitude may include:

- *Refining* – modest adjustments in the way work is carried out.
- *Rectifying* – correcting and remedying problems and failures.
- *Constructing* – extending scope and scale of the service through collaboration with other groups and agencies.

- *Building* – increasing strength and power through resource development.
- *Transforming* – fundamentally changing the way work is done.

It is probable that frontline healthcare professionals may reasonably exploit more opportunities in the first three levels than the latter two (see Boxes 11.1 and 11.2) and opportunities for middle managers are likely to reduce between 'refining' and 'transforming'. As Darzi (2007: 15) acknowledges, it is at these basic levels that 'staff can see that changes need to be made. They now need the space to act on this'.

Bruhn (2004: 135) argues that change leaders should use strategies appropriate to their organizations' stages in the life-cycle. He suggests that creative change is relevant for new organizations but mature organizations respond better to 'managed' or planned change. Burnes (1996: 16) agrees, arguing that bureaucratic 'role' cultures (see Chapter 8) appear to have a closer alignment with the planned model of change. On the other hand, 'task' cultures (see below) tend to promote ends over means and are associated with a more flexible, decentralized style of management and appear more in tune with emergent models of change (see Chapter 6). Burnes (1996: 16) summarizes that it is therefore 'difficult to see how an organization with a "role" culture could easily or successfully adopt the decentralized and participative procedures of the emergent models'.

This position, discussed in more detail in the next section, causes difficulties for policy makers, planners and managers when introducing change in the mature 'role' cultures found in healthcare.

In discussing change in healthcare, Davies et al. (2000: 115) claim that strategies for cultural change should be selective, aiming for a balance between continuity and renewal, identifying those cultural aspects to keep and reinforce and those which should be renewed. Harvey-Jones argues:

> The more complicated the management problems, the more there is a need for a simple, clear statement of strategy which is first and foremost achievable and acceptable but which is also comprehensible to everyone who works in the organization – go back to first principles. (Harvey-Jones, 1990: 137)

These 'first principles' include:

- A belief in and use of evidence.
- Centrality of patient care.
- A commitment to quality.
- Awareness of the constraints imposed by external influences on cultural values, especially those arising from the various healthcare professions.
- The needs, fears and motivations of staff at all levels.
  (Davies et al., 2000)

Balfour and Clarke (2001) caution that strategies should not be at the expense of the change content itself and Rushmer et al. (2004a: 402) argue that strategy development must emanate from within the group itself and not be imposed from outside (see Box 11.1).

Culture and structure

The bureaucratic cultures and structures of healthcare organizations have been discussed in Chapters 7 and 8. Cultural beliefs and practices are perpetuated through:

1 Professional training and post-registration educational programmes.
2 Methods of induction, mentoring, clinical supervision and individual appraisals.
3 Working to specific job descriptions and performance criteria.

In relation to change management, Handy (1993: 186) describes 'role' culture organizations, typically found in healthcare, as 'slow to perceive the need for change and slow to change even if the need is seen'. For frontline practitioners to be enabled to be innovative and meet the policy objectives of implementing change these conditions have to be radically altered and replaced by:

- Flexible structures characterized by decentralization.
- Strategies emphasizing shared decision making.
- Reduced but moderate use of formal rules and regulation.
- More broadly defined job descriptions.
- Flexible lines of authority with fewer hierarchical levels.
  (Martins and Terblanche, 2003)

In contrast to 'role' cultures, Handy (1993) describes 'task' cultures as reflecting qualities which:

- focus on getting a job done;
- are based on expert power (rather than position or person power);
- cultivate a team culture with wide influence;
- are created for specific tasks;
- contain decision-making powers;
- are judged by results;
- have a high level of group control.

Regarding managing change, Handy (1993: 188–9) sees 'task' or 'team' culture as being extremely adaptable, flexible, creative and quick to react and is 'the culture most in tune with current ideologies of change and adaptation'.

Martins and Terblanche (2003: 70) indicate that where there is a flat structure and greater autonomy in work teams, innovation will be promoted. This is in contrast to inhibiting factors of formalization, standardization and centralization (see Chapter 3). As indicated in the fundamental principles above 'the values of flexibility as opposed to rigidity and freedom as opposed to control' are emphasized throughout the change literature.

Changing culture or changing structure

One of the key debates in change management literature revolves around whether behaviour change is achieved through focusing on culture or structure. Chapter 7 outlined how group and organizational culture influence the development of structures but explains that over time (as in mature organizations) structures come to dominate, limit and control work methods and routines and become the 'primary culture-creating mechanisms' that constrain and control employees' behaviour (Schein, 2004: 262). Attempts to effect behaviour change in healthcare historically focus on changing beliefs and values through stressing new visions, mission statements and 'culture change' training programmes (Davies et al., 2000; DH, 2000a; 2004a). Beer et al. (1990: 159) argue that this is the 'fallacy of programmatic change'. This is because change programmes are based on the false belief that if attitudes and values are changed behavioural change will follow. Beer et al. state that this theory gets the change process back to front and indicates why change-training programmes do not produce any change. Eccles (1994) argues that changing shared values is probably the most complex and least understood type of change but changing the culture before implementing a strategic drive is a sub-optimal method. He is quite clear about the focus of activity and how the sequence of events should unfold:

> In the argument about the relative importance of culture, the chicken and egg concern has been whether you could alter behaviour and performance without first having a cultural change, or whether the culture changes when you make organizational alterations. As soon as you pose the dilemma, the answer becomes clear. How could you change the culture while the work goes on as before in an unchanged organization? In the absence of a driving force – a need to change which cannot be ignored – why should the culture change? What, to the organization's inhabitants, would be the point of adopting different beliefs if there is no apparent goal apart from that of changing for change's sake? (Eccles, 1994: 211)

Hendry (1996) and Beer et al. (1990) stress that by putting people into new roles and new structures with new responsibilities and relationships their behaviour will be channelled in new and different directions. Hendry (1996: 633) claims that 'behaviour has therefore to change before a new or modified value system can become a reality'. As the strategic shift unfolds and staff deal with the mental disruption caused by new learning so the culture will change (Eccles, 1994). As new behaviours are tried out and found to be effective so new attitudes and assumptions will emerge and embed the lessons learnt in the culture (Carroll and Quijada, 2004).

What are the optimum strategies available to managers to cater for this in the 'role' culture of healthcare? The strategy would be to create a 'task' culture *within* the organizational role culture. Whether these are termed 'semi-autonomous groups', 'communities of practice', 'action learning sets', 'co-researchers', 'task' or 'ad hoc team structures' they all share key concepts in the furtherance of change (Hendry, 1996: 634–5; Padaki, 2002: 327–8):

- Project-based work carried out in groups and sub-groups stressing social learning.
- Emphasis on 'services' rather than products.

- Emphasis on problem solving which enhances organizational capability.
- 'Interdisciplinary' tasks with strong inter-dependencies in roles and functions.
- Encouragement of cross-group and cross-project interdependencies.
- Concurrent learning and doing – this indicates an emphasis on adult learning theory and action research approaches.
- Small changes in variance such as changing desks, offices or team roles and responsibilities can create experiential learning and a more positive perspective on change.
- Introduction of an ongoing cycle of change through work and team rotation.

Job rotation, for example, increases the technical skill and range of group members' activities through multi-skilling which broadens their understanding and appreciation of the 'whole task' and increases quality (Dunphy and Bryant, 1996: 687). Orgland (1997) argues that 'problem-solving teams' can be made more permanent to emulate the Japanese concept of *kaizen*, the creation of a culture of sustained continuous improvement similar to Wallis and Tyson's (2003) study in Box 11.2.

Box 11.2

Overview

Wallis and Tyson (2003) report on a study concerning an action research project to improve the management and care of patients in a Hematology/Oncology Day Unit in Australia. The demand for the service increased causing reduction in care standards (patient waiting, symptom management and patient education) and increases in complaints.

Initial exploratory and fact-finding phase

- Staff meetings held.
- Incident reports and patient complaints examined.
- Clinical staff observed.
- Historically, staff complement was set by service episodes rather than chemotherapy protocols; staff were either under-used or very busy and had insufficient time for counselling or education.

Decision and action phase 1

- A multi-disciplinary group of oncologists, pharmacists and nurses devised and regularly updated a 'chemotherapy protocol manual' detailing treatment needs to enable a more accurate timescale for patient care and a realistic, timed appointment system.
- Protocol included: assessment, pharmacy and set-up time; type of chemotherapy regimen, personnel and equipment needs.
- Common patient records used by all multi-disciplinary team members.

(Continued)

(Continued)

Nurses thought there were still inefficiencies and further plans were made to improve appointment and staff allocation systems.

Phase 2 fact-finding

- Over three months, pre-intervention and post-intervention data around chemotherapy including: infection rates, drug errors, accuracy of protocols.
- Treatment times were collected from records, incident reports, infection control and pharmacy databases.
- Patient satisfaction data collected via completion of anonymous survey pre- and post-intervention, three months apart, including: overall experience, waiting and appointment time, staff communication and professionalism, overall symptom management and control.
- Open-ended questions regarding opportunities to improve service.

Decision and action phase 2

- Data analysed descriptively and qualitatively.
- Selected findings post-intervention: delays reduced from 111.5 hrs to 77 hrs; prescription accuracy problems reduced from seven to five (doctors) and four to three (nurses).
- Patient satisfaction post-intervention improved from 40.8 to 42.24 (max score 45).
- Lowest ranked items pre-intervention: waiting time and education talk.
- Highest ranked items: staff courtesy and professionalism.

Items of importance to patients were education, being comfortable and able to relax and having faith in the service and staff.
   Actions taken:

1   Redesign appointment system to enable even spread over day.
2   'Primary caregiver' allocated for specific patients at beginning of day.
3   Set up 'review clinic' for non-treatment patients.
4   Computer-based 'chart requesting system' for review and treatment clinic set up.
5   Application for unit's refurbishment to promote patient comfort was granted.

Phase 3 fact-finding

- Data collected similarly to Phase 2 but focused on second-worst ranked 'patient education'.
- Data collected via survey on patient knowledge of symptoms, treatment, medications, their side-effects and use of cancer support services.

Decision and action phase 3

Actions aimed at increasing primary nursing, matching patient need with nurse capability:

- Staff training focused on patient education and information-giving strategies.
- Staff meetings to assess impact.

Evaluation

Pre- and post-implementation test results:

- More patients able to record answers to questions.
- Patients still saw doctors and nurses as key support and advice givers.
- Indications of referral to cancer services increased slightly.
- Applications to Cancer Fund increased from 18 to 40.
- Referrals to dietitian decreased. Referrals to social workers increased.

Summary

Further improvements are planned around involving peripheral staff (dietitians, social workers, psychologists) in day-to-day patient care to emphasize their contribution and improve prophylaxis and care. Changing the appointment system increased time available for psychosocial care by nurses.

The elucidation of these strategies implies a reframing of approaches to leadership.

Leadership

Here concepts from the 'co-ordinate' ovoid (Figure 4.1) are considered. As argued in Chapter 5, consistent research has shown that the most effective leadership style is one in which the leader/manager shares power with subordinates. This style increases both the satisfaction and effectiveness of followers, in other words the most effective leaders are those who are able to cede power to their staff (Huczynski and Buchanan, 2001).

Padaki (2002: 329–30) argues that to be effective, managers and leaders must transform:

- From authoritative to facilitative leadership. This will broaden the power-base for decision-making (Timpson, 1998: 264).
- From vertical to multi-lateral accountability including leader to group accountability.
- From manipulative to collaborative orientation.

Padaki explains that the entire discipline of organizational change and improvement rests on democratic, egalitarian and humanistic values. He claims that 'if managers and leaders do not find these acceptable then no progress will be made' (2002: 325).

Empowerment can be threatening to some leaders which they may see as diminishing their own powerbase. They therefore need to feel secure enough to allow their staff to take control (Johnson, 1998: 145). Martins and Terblanche (2003) argue that a facilitative role for managers and leaders implies that they outline a set of strategic goals as guidelines but allow their staff freedom of implementation within the context of the goals. This is a position supported by Darzi (2007: 16) who argues that systems should 'support local change from the centre rather than instructing it'.

In their extensive report into the effectiveness of healthcare teams, Borrill et al. (2001) show that where there is no clear leader or co-ordinator or where there is conflict over leadership, team objectives will be unclear producing low levels of participation, low commitment to quality and support leading to low levels of effectiveness and innovation. A similar report by the Royal Pharmaceutical Society (2000: 33) recommends that leaders are selected on the basis of their leadership skills rather than on the basis of status, hierarchy or availability (see Chapter 5).

Managers need to resist the temptation to intervene, over manage, overreact, and protect the team from responsibility. Instead they need to become better listeners, facilitators and coaches without abdicating their managerial responsibility (Eccles, 1994). Managers make better decisions when they take soundings from their staff who have practical experience of the work. The leadership role is therefore flexible dependent on the application of expertise at the required time. This reflects Follett's contention of the 'leadership of function' (Fox and Urwick, 1973: 282) where those with knowledge and skills are enabled to manage the situation. But this does not imply a relegation of responsibility by managers who should have a goal to achieve but not a blueprint. Eccles (1994) describes it as the dialogue in a classic Western film where followers ask 'Which way should we go' and receive the answer 'Go West'. The destination is clear: the route is flexible.

Rogers (1983) outlines the characteristics of two modes of teaching which can be translated into strategies for successful change management (indeed Follett (Fox and Urwick, 1973: 232) notes the American Management Association's members' 'conviction that "leader" and "teacher" are synonymous terms'.)

The 'traditional' mode

- The manager is the possessor of knowledge/power, the worker the recipient.
- Command is the major method of getting the worker to act.
- Reports and appraisals measure the extent to which work has been achieved.
- The manager is the possessor of power, the worker the one who obeys.
- Trust is at a minimum: notably the manager's distrust of the worker.
- Democratic values are ignored in practice: the worker does not participate in choosing the aims, the product or the manner of working.

The politics of traditional management are clear. Decisions are made at the top. 'Power over' is an important position and monitoring, control and supervision are key concepts.

The 'person-centred' mode

- The precondition is for leaders who are sufficiently secure within themselves and their relationships with others that they experience an essential trust in the capacity of others to think and learn for themselves.

- Facilitative managers and leaders share responsibility for the change process with team members.
- Managers and leaders provide structure, support and resources, from within themselves and their experience. The team develops its own schedule of work.
- The focus is primarily on fostering the continuing process of learning while working: 'A course is successfully ended not when the student has "learned all she needs to know" but when she has made significant progress in learning how to learn what she wants to know' (Rogers, 1983: 189).
- The evaluation of the extent and significance of team learning is made primarily by the members.
- In this 'growth-promoting' work climate, learning tends to be deeper, proceeds at a more rapid rate, and is more pervasive in life and behaviour than learning acquired in the traditional mode.
- The direction is guided or self-chosen, the learning is self-initiated and the whole person (with feelings and passions as well as intellect) is invested in the process.

The politics of the 'person-centred' mode

Rogers considers the political implications: who has the essential power and control? It is clear that it is the staff members. Who is attempting to gain control over whom? The staff are in the process of gaining control over the course of their own work. The manager relinquishes control over others, retaining only control over her or himself.

Communication

Here the concepts from the ovoids 'communicate' and 'consult' (Figure 4.1) are considered.

Burnes (2004: 480) asserts that communication is not just informing staff that change is being considered, but should involve them in discussions and debates about the need for, and form of, change and allow them the freedom to discuss the issues involved openly and without fear of censure. He argues that there needs to be clear and persuasive arguments for the change, and gaining the backing and support of all staff and stakeholders gives strength to the project. Beer and Eisenstat (1996) call for open discussion of all aspects of the process; if teams lack the capacity for open discussion they cannot arrive at a shared diagnosis, if they lack a diagnosis they cannot agree on an end state nor a strategy to achieve it.

Brooks and Brown (2002) suggest that a useful strategy to demonstrate a need for change is to carry out external 'fact-finding' visits which serve to challenge existing practices and can legitimize changes. They describe managers taking staff away to view other, similar workplaces as the only way to get them to see opportunities for themselves (see Box 8.2).

Potter et al. (1994) discuss an action research project to facilitate continuous quality management in three departments in a district general hospital. Staff visited the operating theatres in another hospital to raise interest, develop teamwork and to help reflect on their work. The strategy was very positive in forwarding change with increased contentment, reflection and plans to reorganize areas such as scheduling, equipment layout and use of uniforms. However, the Operating Department Assistants noted that, contrary to their practice, medical staff cleaned their own boots. On their return they persuaded the theatre manager to change this practice causing consternation and conflict among their medical colleagues.

Pettigrew (1979: 578) points out that language is one of the key tools of social influence and that leaders' effectiveness is likely to be influenced by the language overlap with their followers and by the extent to which a leader can create words that explain and thereby give order to collective experience. Brooks and Brown (2002) give examples of simply changing staff nomenclature from 'domestic staff' to 'care assistant' which was seen as inclusive, bringing them into the wider ward team where they felt more valued.

Alternatively, poor explanation and communication can result in mistrust and apprehension regarding role encroachment and a lack of understanding of other professions (Royal Pharmaceutical Society, 2000: 18).

Participation

Here concepts from the ovoid 'collaborate' (Figure 4.1) are considered.

Participation, seen as 'the greater involvement of workers under conditions of openness, trust and free exchange' (Orgland, 1997: 197) is one of the core change principles and the overwhelming strategy of choice for managing resistance (Waddell and Sohal, 1998). In the first study examining resistance (see Chapter 9), Coch and French (1947) argue that participation was the primary method to overcome it. Eccles (1994) claims that as a strategic method it is most appropriate for professional and collegial organizations where a manager's or leader's power to intervene would be counter-productive. Carroll and Quijada (2004:ii17) found that the change process has more chance to succeed if key individuals are involved in the planning and design of interventions that solve real problems, since this process engages and satisfies their internal motivation – they therefore become committed rather than simply compliant (Waddell and Sohal, 1998). Parkin (1999b) argues that research has consistently shown that individuals' participation in implementing change builds ownership, motivates success and reduces resistance. Orgland argues participation's real merit is that:

> It can generate new ideas, make it possible for these ideas to be taken advantage of, connect people to the definition and solution of problems, increase the likelihood that people's capabilities are utilized and improve organizational performance. (Orgland, 1997: 198)

As Padaki (2002: 331) argues, the group itself 'must conceive, design, plan, implement, and manage the operating system involved in the change process'.

Bridges and Meyer's study shows a health service manager's frustration with the Trust when senior staff are not consulted:

They're used to having the expert at the top, you know the information comes in from outside, the experts decide how to deal with [it] and then they tell the troops what to do, whereas in an organization in my mind the experts are actually at the bottom because they're the ones doing the work, the clinicians etc, but they were not consulted, how can we change an organization without consulting anybody. (Bridges and Meyer, 2007: 396)

In their study to assess the effects of head nurses' leadership styles on their staff's levels of emotional exhaustion, Stordeur et al. (2001) report that managers and leaders who allow employees greater participation in decision-making and encouraged a two-way communication process tended to generate a favourable climate among their nursing team. This was characterized by less interpersonal conflict, less hostility and fewer non-cooperative relationships. They also showed that clearly assigning tasks, specifying procedures, and clarifying expectations result in reduced role ambiguity and increased job satisfaction among employees.

Concerning resistance, Dent and Powley (2002) report in their study of 239 employees who had experienced, cumulatively, nearly 1,000 change events, that responders were more likely to view change positively if they had initiated or taken part in implementation. Conversely those who responded negatively typically did not actively participate or completely understand the change project.

Encouraging and facilitating participation leads to enhanced possibilities for team learning, however there can be significant drawbacks, particularly around the time involved in the participative process.

Team learning

The importance of innovation being team-centred has been emphasized in Chapters 5, 7 and 8. Schein (2004) argues that change will only be achieved when the emphasis is placed on teams rather than individuals.

Rushmer et al. (2004b: 377) stress that encouraging and focusing on team learning builds flexibility, produces multiple levels of responsiveness, reduces dependency on key staff, opens up work systems to new ideas and reduces the need for a strong managerial push. Ferlie and Shortell (2001: 284) found that strategies to improve quality which focus on individuals are seldom effective. They argue that group-based approaches reinforce the team microcosm, help build greater understanding among members and spread leadership practices more rapidly than programmes aimed at each person separately. In this way teams contribute to organizational learning as shown in Figure 8.1.

Self-managing teams tend to be associated with better performance because self-management increases members' responsibilities and ownership of the work (Ferlie and Shortell, 2001: 295), increases job satisfaction and promotes a better quality of life (Dunphy and Bryant, 1996).

Borrill et al. (2001) and Dunphy and Bryant (1996) note that teamwork is better suited to promote innovation than individual arrangements. This is particularly relevant in responding to ever changing customer demands for new, improved services. This occurs in the study in Box 11.2, when a wider range of skills, knowledge and experience results in more perspectives and solutions for solving client problems.

The Royal Pharmaceutical Society (2000: 18) and Borrill et al. (2001) report factors which promote teamwork and collaboration. These occur where:

- Members share vision, values and philosophy.
- Team members' roles and responsibilities are seen as essential, are clearly understood, and there are clear team goals.
- There is effective communication and optimum team size.
- There is mutual recognition of team members' professional judgement and discretion.
- There is a climate of reflective learning.
- Adequate time and resources are ensured.
- A shared learning process pervades.

Apart from 'time' these criteria are evident in Galvin et al.'s study in Box 11.1. Thorne (1997: 178) claims that collegial and professional cultures which operate as networks or flatter structures and are designed to empower and support rather than control, are likely to be the most effective organizational configurations.

Edge and Laiken (2002) and Borrill et al. (2001) note that team performance is most effective when rewards are administered to the team as a whole and not to individuals, and when they provide incentives for collaboration and communication rather than individualized work. This reinforces individuals working together as a team. Yet, they argue, in healthcare, teamwork is undermined where, for example, bonus payments are paid to GPs as part of their independent contractor status, despite the whole team contributing to final outcomes.

Dunphy and Bryant (1996) also note their research which found that in the public sector centralized team structures prevailed. They propose that reasons could be related to the traditional bureaucratic organizational model and that self-managing teams may be too threatening to basic values.

Conclusion

Writing in 1993, Nicholson notes the paradox of change. On the one hand most organizations aim, rightfully, to create stability, order and continuity for the working lives of their staff and those who use their services or buy their products. On the other, they are under constant pressure, both internally and externally, to evolve and improve their quality and performance to ensure their own and their employees' survival. Despite organizations' need and desire to change, a 'dynamic conservatism' means they absorb, neutralize or even reverse the attempts of their employees to innovate. Hence Nicholson (1993: 210) argues that because individual change agents are confronted by the 'difficult and dangerous task of challenging fundamental assumptions … top-down, rather than bottom-up, approaches to intervention are necessary to implement radical change'. This rationale conflicts with more recent analyses and the position taken in this text which views this as inappropriate. Reasons for this include the move from 'the "controlling" to the "involving" paradigm' (Dunphy and Bryant, 1996: 692) and the development of group approaches to change through action research and communities of practice which can offer greater support to individuals through the inherent expansion of leadership practices, knowledge and skills, and the social support of multiple voices.

Chapter summary

- There is a vast array of change implementation strategies ranging from authoritarian coercion to full partnership of equals.
- The optimum strategy for change in professional organizations is to build consensus and ownership through participation and education.
- Team-based rather than individual-based strategies are more effective in creating and framing opportunities for change.
- Strategies creating participation and involvement are time and labour intensive.

12

Conclusions

This book is about managing change in healthcare. The policy message is simple – where there is need to introduce a new local service, make improvements to an existing service or solve a problem which develops patient and client care – just do it. But seeing change as simple does not make it straightforward. Implementing lasting change is not easy.

The book is written against a backdrop of a world occupied by increasingly complex problems. These problems not only relate to the complexity of modern health and disease, its treatment, care and management but also to healthcare organizations, the costs and administration of their services, their management and leadership and, perhaps most significantly, the politics governing them. Not only this, but the social and global environment is changing rapidly, driven by:

- technological advances that do not necessarily contribute to facilitating better service provision;
- rising consumer demands;
- the current political imperative of providing choice;
- increased costs triggering Treasury restrictions on treatments and services.

These forces can give health services the appearance of seriously lagging behind events and expectations in the wider world.

For the purpose of analysis and ease of explication, the many and varied phenomena of change are organized discretely into chapters to provide 'frameworks of understanding' (Dunphy, 1996: 542).

However, in the reality of changing practice all these phenomena will overlap and run concurrently. Instigators of change will:

- assess their organizational context (to a greater or lesser extent);
- develop some sort of plan (whether this is termed an 'approach' or 'process' hardly matters);
- apply knowledge, skills and ideas drawn from management and leadership theory (whether they are deemed managers, leaders, practitioners or change agents hardly matters);

- be imbued with many of their organizations' and professional groups' cultural beliefs and practices which may limit their clarity of purpose, opportunities and effectiveness;
- draw from a compendium of implementation strategies ranging from authoritarian coercion to the educationally participative.

But from where does the impetus for change – to create, improve, develop, and progress healthcare practice, emerge?

Asking questions

The triggers for change come from discomfort.

Where there is comfort, complacency and satisfaction, change will not happen and, when change attempts are made, they will be resisted.

At all levels of professional education, the development of a critical approach must be fostered. As Bauman (1990: 18) states, 'to encourage critical scrutiny of beliefs hitherto uncritically held; to promote a habit of self-analysis and of questioning the views that pretend to be certainties'; only through this can the familiar become defamiliarized.

Implementing change

Implicit in the term in-NOVA-tion is something new rather than something different. Implementing change is always difficult but the tightening of practice guidelines restricts real innovation and taxes the most resourceful and determined practitioner. Individuals alone cannot achieve institutional change and though the philosophy of current health policy may, rightly, be empowerment and delegation of decision-making (DH, 2000a), and

> Even though 'managing change' has become one of nursing's articles of faith and because managers and educators value and desire practitioners who are innovative, it can not be assumed that innovation will be the hallmark of their work (Parkin, 1997: 139).

This is because what politicians promise on the one hand through the rhetoric of empowerment and devolution of decision-making, they take away through increased centralized control, the micromanagement of actions, the imposition of top-down targets devised far away from the delivery of care and a focus on the individual worker rather than the system as a whole.

Rose, a GP, reacts: 'I am increasingly frustrated in my professional role by being told what I can and, perhaps more importantly, cannot do. Guidelines and edicts from important bodies rain upon me' (Rose, 2005: 16).

The tyranny of targets

The politicization of health has led to the belief that politicians only value what can be measured (as spurious evidence of achievement) and that if something needs to be done, then the way to achievement is to re-create it as a target (with penalties for non-achievement). Measurement can then be published in league tables (to name and shame), for the wider electorate as proof of success (or failure); hence, there is an over-concentration on achieving targets. The focus of practice therefore is born out of the conception of targets. Thus, to get things done, everything must be a target, resulting in accusations of micromanagement. Clinical expertise and leadership (the very qualities the politicians claim they value), are expropriated to the state.

The fallacy of leadership?

Leadership, collaboration and learning will not grow in such an environment. Staff should be freed from the monolithic organizational structures, the cultural straitjackets of professional boundaries and the tyranny of governmental targets. Rushmer et al. (2004b) argue that all recent health reforms have been top-down and externally imposed. This offers little autonomy, thwarts the discretion of expert practitioners, creates resistance and indifference and restricts organizational learning. Ministers and executives must have more confidence and trust in the ability of frontline staff to see local opportunities and manage them through appropriate actions. As Dunphy argues (1996: 551) 'there is an uneasy tension between executive level strategic direction and intelligent, committed and innovative action on the part of the ... workforce'.

The 'great-man' theory, an out-dated concept of leadership, has to pass. Leadership is not about authority, oration or control but functional leaders who can cross territorial boundaries, integrate staff's experience and expertise and use it for a common purpose.

But how can functional leadership be employed to manage change?

Why action research?

Burgess-Macey and Rose (1997: 62) make a robust case for action research as a significant vehicle for professional development particularly in situations where professionals suffer from low status, are de-professionalized, disenfranchised, feel powerless and are marginalized by government policies. They claim that professionals are able to regain their status, integrity and self-esteem through action research, as projects are:

- voluntary rather than imposed;
- focused on their own research rather then being directed by management;
- within their own control rather than following prescribed formats;
- evaluated by themselves or research partners rather than by external inspectorates;

- undertaken in safe and supportive environments rather than in cultures of blame and criticism;
- adapted to suit the needs, demands and pace of their work settings rather than an additional burden within a hard-pressed timetable;
- able to provide contexts for practitioners' own voice;
- able to create contexts for critical self-enquiry.

Action research, therefore, represents a powerful challenge to the status quo with its scrutiny of entrenched culture-based structures, practices and opinions; real worker empowerment becomes a viable means to implement change.

A school careers officer fed back to Greenhalgh et al.'s (2006: 4–6) study (Box 7.1): 'it is to your eternal credit that you turned talk into action. I've helped out a lot of people with research projects and most of it never leads to anything'.

Deery (2005: 165) also notes that in the troubled culture of midwifery, the metaphor of giving 'voice' to a group with a history of being ignored was vital in providing the opportunity to reflect on deeply entrenched negative attitudes and enable growth. Action research incorporates direct worker participation in the strategic planning process and, stressing an evolutionary approach through a cyclical model (Figure 6.5), becomes a vehicle to integrate education, research and practice development. As Rahnema (1990) agues: 'Long-term and serious processes of social and individual transformations are, essentially, the work of small groups of individuals awakened to the world to which they relate' (cited in Pyrch, 2007: 210).

Ultimately, achieving meaningful change that benefits patients and enables staff and organizational learning is best managed through the integration and collaboration of expert, frontline staff themselves. This is the pinnacle of professional practice.

References

Adair, J. (2004), *The John Adair Handbook of Management and Leadership* (N. Thomas, ed.). London: Thorogood.

Albritton, R. and Shaughnessy, T. (1990), *Developing Leadership Skills.* Englewood, CO: Libraries Unlimited Inc.

Albrow, M. (ed.) (1990), *Globalization, Knowledge and Society.* London: Sage.

Alderson, P. (1998), Theories in health care and research – the importance of theories in health care, *British Medical Journal*, 317 (7164), 1007–10.

Alimo-Metcalfe, B. (1996), Leaders or Managers? *Nursing Management*, 3(1), 22–4.

Alimo-Metcalfe, B. and Alban-Metcalfe, J. (2003), Stamp of Greatness, *Health Service Journal*, 26 June, 113 (5861), 28–31.

Alimo-Metcalfe, B. and Lawler, J. (2001), Leadership development in UK companies at the beginning of the twenty-first century: lessons for the NHS? *Journal of Management in Medicine*, 15 (5), 387–404.

Altrichter, H., Kemmis, S., McTaggart, R. and Zuber-Skerritt, O. (2002), The concept of action research, *The Learning Organization*, 9 (3), 125–31.

Amitay, M., Popper, M. and Lipshitz, R. (2005), Leadership styles and organizational learning in community clinics, *The Learning Organization*, 12 (1), 57–70.

Ancona, D., Malone, T., Orlikowski, W. and Senge, P. (2007), In praise of the incomplete leader, *Harvard Business Review*, 85 (2), 92–100.

Anderson, E. (2005), Approaches to conflict resolution, *British Medical Journal*, 331 (7512), 344–6.

Appleyard, B. (2002), Leaders of the pack, *Sunday Times*, 20 January.

Appleyard, B. (2005), The maverick art of leadership, *Sunday Times*, 9 January.

Argyris, C. and Schon, D. (1978), *Organizational Learning.* Reading, MA: Addison-Wesley.

Aronson, J.K., Henderson, G., Webb, D.J. and Rawlins, M.D. (2006), A prescription for better prescribing, *British Medical Journal*, 333 (7566), 459–60.

Ashford, J., Eccles, M., Bond, S., Hall, L. and Bond, J. (1999), Improving health care through professional behaviour change: introducing a framework for identifying behaviour change strategies, *British Journal of Clinical Governance*, 4 (1), 14–23.

Attwood, M. and Beer, N. (1988), Development of a learning organisation – reflections on a personal and organisational workshop in a District Health Authority, *Management Education and Development*, 19 (3), 201–14.

Avery, G. (2004), *Understanding Leadership*. London: Sage.

Badger, T.G. (2000), Action research: change and methodological rigour, *Journal of Nursing Research*, 8 (4), 201–7.

Baggott, R. (2004), *Health and Health Care in Britain*, 3rd edn. Basingstoke: Palgrave Macmillan.

Bagshaw, M. (1998), Conflict management and mediation: key leadership skills for the millennium, *Industrial and Commercial Training*, 30 (6), 206–8.

Baldridge, J. and Deal, T. (1975), Overview of change processes in educational organizations. In: J. Baldridge and T. Deal. (eds), *Managing Change in Educational Organizations: Sociological Perspectives*. Berkeley: Cutchan Press, pp. 1–23.

Balfour, M. and Clarke, C. (2001), Searching for sustainable change, *Journal of Clinical Nursing*, 10, 44–50.

Bamford, D. and Forrester, P. (2003), Managing planned and emergent change within an operations management environment, *International Journal of Operations and Production Management*, 23 (5), 546–64.

Bass, B. (1990), *Bass and Stogdill's Handbook of Leadership: Theory, Research, and Managerial Application*, 3rd edn. New York: Free Press.

Bate, P. (2000), Synthesizing research and practice: Using the action research approach in health care settings, *Social Policy and Administration*, 34 (4), 478–93.

Bauman, Z. (1990), *Thinking Sociologically*. Oxford: Blackwell.

Beer, M. and Eisenstat, R. (1996), Developing an organization capable of implementing strategy and learning, *Human Relations*, 49 (5), 597–619.

Beer, M., Eisenstat, R. and Spencer, B. (1990), Why change programmes don't produce change, *Harvard Business Review*, Nov/Dec, 158–66.

Belbin, M. (1981), *Management Teams – Why they Succeed or Fail*. London: Heineman.

Bennett, B. (1998), Increasing collaboration within a multidisciplinary neurohabilitation team: the early stages of a small action research project, *Journal of Clinical Nursing*, 7, 227–31.

Bennis, W. and Nanus, B. (1985), *Leaders: The Strategies for Taking Charge*, New York: Harper and Row.

Bencit, C. and Mackensie, K. (1994), A model of organizational learning and the diagnostic process supporting it, *The Learning Organization*, 1 (3), 26–37.

Berge, B.-M. (2001), Action research for gender equity in a late modern society, *International Journal of Inclusive Education*, 5 (2/3), 281–92.

Berwick, D., Ham, C. and Smith, R., (2003), Would the NHS benefit from a single, identifiable leader? An email conversation, *British Medical Journal*, 327 (7429), 1421–4.

Betts, J. and Holden, R. (2003), Organisational learning in a public sector organisation: a case study in muddled thinking, *Journal of Workplace Learning*, 15 (6), 280–7.

Blair, A. (2005), Jamie's dinners push healthy school food up political menu, *The Times*, 19 March.

Blair, T. (2002), *The Courage of our Convictions: Why Reform of the Public Services is the Route to Social Justice*. London: Fabian Society.

211

Blake, R. and Mouton, J. (1964), *The Managerial Grid*. Houston: Gulf Publishing.

Blane, D. (1997), Health professions. In: G. Scambler (ed.), *Sociology as Applied to Medicine*, 4th edn. London: W.B. Saunders Company Ltd, pp. 212–24.

Blau, P. and Scott, W. (1963), *Formal Organizations: A Comparative Approach*. London: Routledge & Kegan Paul.

Bohmer, R. and Edmonson, A. (2001), Organizational learning in health care, *Health Forum Journal*, March/April, 32–5.

Bolton, S. (2003), Multiple roles?: nurses as managers in the NHS, *The International Journal of Public Sector Management*, 16 (2), 122–30.

Bolton, S. (2004), A simple matter of control? NHS hospital nurses and new management, *Journal of Management Studies*, 41 (2), 317–33.

Bone, J. (2003), UN chief will not break protocol, *The Times*, 28 March.

Borrill, C., Carletta, J., Carter, A., Dawson, J., Garrod, S., Rees, A., Richards, A., Shapiro. D. and West, M. (2001), *The Effectiveness of Health Care Teams in the National Health Service*, Birmingham: Aston University.

Bradshaw, P. (2002), Managers, blame culture and highly ambitious policies in the British National Health Service (NHS), *Journal of Nursing Management*, 10, 1–4.

Brazier, D.K. (2005), Influence of contextual factors on health-care leadership, *Leadership and Organization Development Journal*, 6 (2), 128–40.

Brearley, M. (2000), Teams: lessons from the world of sport, *British Medical Journal*, 321, 1141–3.

Bridges, J. and Meyer, J. (2007), Exploring the effectiveness of action research as a tool for organizational change in health care, *Journal of Research in Nursing*, 12 (4), 389–99.

British Medical Association (BMA) (2007), 'Flawed' government plans on urgent care overlook GPs, BMA warns (issued 2 February 2007) http://www.bma.org.uk/pressrel.nsf/wlu/SGOY6XZEG3?OpenDocument&vw=wfmms (accessed 5 April 2007).

Brooks, C. (2006), Working with healthcare professionals. In: K. Walshe and J. Smith (eds), *Healthcare Management*. Maidenhead: Open University Press, pp. 253–68.

Brooks, I. and Brown, R.B. (2002), The role of ritualistic ceremonial in removing barriers between subcultures in the National Health Service, *Journal of Advanced Nursing*, 38 (4), 341–52.

Brooten, D., Hayman, L. and Naylor, M. (1978), *Leadership for change: A guide for the frustrated nurse*. New Jersey: Prentice Hall.

Brown, A. (1998), *Organizational Culture*, 2nd edn. London: Pitman.

Brown, T. and Jones, L. (2001), *Action Research and Postmodernism: Congruence and Critique*. Buckingham: Open University Press.

Bruce, R. and Wyman, S. (1998), *Changing Organizations: Practicing Action Training and Research*. Thousand Oaks: Sage Publications.

Bruhn. J. (2004), Leaders who create change and those who manage it: how leaders limit success, *The Health Care Manager*, 23 (2), 132–40.

Buchanan, D. and Badham, R. (1999), *Power, Politics, and Organizational Change: Winning the Turf Game*. London: Sage Publications.

Buchanan, D., Fitzgerald, L., Ketley, D., Gollop, R., Jones, J.L., Lamont, S.S., Neath, A. and Whitby, E. (2005), No going back: A review of the literature on sustaining organizational change, *International Journal of Management Reviews*, 7 (3), 189–205.

Burgess-Macey, C. and Rose, J. (1997), Breaking through the barriers: professional development, action research and the early years, *Educational Action Research*, 5 (1), 55–70.

Burnes, B. (1996), No such thing as … a 'one best way' to manage organizational change, *Management Decision*, 34 (10), 11–18.

Burnes, B. (2004), Kurt Lewin and the planned approach to change: a re-appraisal, *Journal of Management Studies*, 41 (6), 977–1002.

Burnes, B., Cooper, C. and West, P. (2003), Organisational learning: the new management paradigm? *Management Decision*, 41 (5), 452–64.

Burns, J. (1978), *Leadership*. New York: Harper & Row.

Butler, S. (2006), Sainsbury's poised to be first supermarket with GP clinics, *The Times*, 10 February.

Cabinet Office (2007), *Capability Review of the Department of Health*. London: Cabinet Office.

Calabrese, R. (2003), The ethical imperative to lead change: overcoming the resistance to change, *The International Journal of Educational Management*, 17 (1), 7–13.

Cameron, I. (2003), Foundation hospitals furore buries threat of surge in GP complaints, *Pulse*, 12 May, 11.

Carroll, J. and Quijada, M. (2004), Redirecting traditional professional values to support safety: Changing organisational culture in health care, *Quality and Safety in Health Care*, 13, supplement 2, ii, 16–21.

Carvel, J. (2005), Record rise in NHS consultants and midwives, *The Guardian*, 23 March.

Chalmers, A. (1999), *What is this Thing Called Science?* 3rd edn. Buckingham: Open University Press.

Chan, A. (1997), Corporate culture of a clan organization, *Management Decision*, 35 (2), 94–9.

Chan, C. (2003), Examining the relationships between individual, team and organizational learning in an Australian hospital, *Learning in Health and Social Care*, 2 (4), 223–35.

Charlton, B. (1993), Medicine and post-modernity, *Journal of the Royal Society of Medicine*, 86, 497–9.

Chin, R. and Benne, K. (1976), General strategies for effective changes in human systems. In: W. Bennis, R. Chin, and K. Corey (eds), *The Planning of Change*, 3rd edn. New York: Holt Rinehart and Winston, pp. 22–45.

Choudrie, J. (2005), Understanding the role of communication and conflict on reengineering team development, *The Journal of Enterprise Information Management*, 18 (1), 64–78.

Chuang, Y.-T., Church, R. and Zikic, J. (2004), Organizational culture, group diversity and intra-group conflict, *Team Performance Management*, 10 (1/2), 26–34.

Coch, L. and French, J. (1947), Overcoming resistance to change, *Human Relations,* 1 (4), 512–32.

Coghlan, D. (1993), A person-centred approach to dealing with resistance to change, *Leadership and Organizational Development Journal,* 14 (4), 10–14.

Coghlan, D. (1994), Managing organizational change through teams and groups, *Leadership and Organizational Development Journal,* 15 (2), 18–23.

Coghlan, D. (2007), Insider action research: opportunities and challenges, *Management Research News,* 30 (5), 335–43.

Coghlan, D. and Brannick, T. (2001), *Doing Action Research in Your Own Organization.* London: Sage.

Coghlan, D. and Casey, M. (2001), Action research from the inside: issues and challenges in doing action research in your own hospital, *Journal of Advanced Nursing,* 35 (5), 674–82.

Cooper, J. and Hewison, A. (2002), Implementing audit in palliative care: an action research approach, *Journal of Advanced Nursing,* 39 (4), 360–9.

Corrigan, P. (2005), *Registering Choice: How Primary Care should Change to Meet Patients' Needs.* London: Social Market Foundation.

Coughlan, P. and Coghlan, D. (2002), Action research for operations management, *International Journal of Operations and Production Management,* 22 (2), 220–40.

Crozier, M. (1964), *The Bureaucratic Phenomenon.* London: Tavistock Publications.

Cullen, L., Fraser, D. and Symonds, I. (2003), Strategies for interprofessional education: the Interprofessional Team Objective Structured Clinical Examination for midwifery and medical students. *Nurse Education Today,* 23, 427–33.

Currie, G. (1998), Stakeholders' views of management development as a cultural change process in the Health Service. *International Journal of Public Sector Management,* 11 (1), 7–26.

Currie, G. (2000), The role of middle managers in strategic change in the public sector, *Public Money and Management,* Jan–March, 17–22.

Darling, J. and Walker, W. (2001), Effective conflict management: use of the behavioural style model, *Leadership & Organization Development Journal,* 22 (5), 230–42.

Darzi, Professor Lord (2007), *Our NHS our Future – NHS Next Stage Review: Interim Report.* London: Department of Health.

Davidson, D. and Peck, E. (2006), Organizational development and design. In: K. Walshe and J. Smith (eds), *Healthcare Management,* Maidenhead: Open University Press, pp. 342–63.

Davies, C. (1995), *Gender and the Professional Predicament in Nursing.* Buckingham: Open University Press.

Davies, C. (2000), Getting professionals to work together, *British Medical Journal,* 320 (7241), 1021–2.

Davies, H.T.O. and Harrison, S. (2003), Trends in doctor–manager relationships, *British Medical Journal,* 326 (7390), 646–9.

Davies, H.T.O. and Nutley, S. (2000), Developing learning organizations in the new NHS, *British Medical Journal,* 320 998–1001.

Davies, H.T.O., Hodges, C.-L. and Rundall, T. (2003), Views of doctors and managers on the doctor–manager relationship in the NHS, *British Medical Journal,* 326 (7390), 626–8.

Davies, H.T.O., Nutley, S. and Mannion, R. (2000), Organisational culture and quality of health care, *Quality in Health Care*, 9, 111–19.

Davis, E. (1997), The leadership role of health services managers, *International Journal of Health Care Quality Assurance incorporating Leadership in Health Services*, 10 (4), i–iv.

Dawson, P. (2003), *Understanding Organizational Change*. London: Sage Publications.

Dean, M. (2003), Battle over foundation hospitals continues, *The Lancet*, 362 (9383), 540–1.

De Dreu, C. (1997), Productive conflict: the importance of conflict management and conflict issue. In: C. De Drew and E. Van de Vliert (eds), *Using Conflict in Organizations*. London: Sage Publications, pp. 9–22.

Deery, R. (2005), An action-research study exploring midwives' support needs and the affect of group clinical supervision, *Midwifery*, 21, 161–76.

Degeling, P. and Carr, A. (2004), Leadership for the systemization of health care: the unaddressed issue in health care reform, *Journal of Health Organization and Management*, 18 (6), 399–414.

Degeling, P., Maxwell, S., Kennedy, J. and Coyle, B. (2003), Medicine, management, and modernization, *British Medical Journal*, 326 (7390), 649–52.

de Jager, P. (2001), Resistance to change: a new view of an old problem, *The Futurist*, May–June, 24–7.

De Loo, I. (2002), The troublesome relationship between action learning and organizational growth, *Journal of Workplace Learning*, 14 (6), 245–55.

Dent, E. and Goldberg, S.G. (1999), Challenging 'resistance to change', *The Journal of Applied Behavioural Science*, 35 (1), 25–41.

Dent, E. and Powley, E. (2002), Employees actually embrace change: The chimera of resistance, *Journal of Applied Management and Entrepreneurship*, 7 (2), 56–73.

Dent, M. (1993), Professionalism, educated labour and the state: hospital medicine and the new managerialism, *The Sociological Review*. 41 (2), 245–73.

Dent, M. (1995), The new National Health Service: a case of postmodernism, *Organization Studies*, 16 (5), 875–99.

Department of Constitutional Affairs (DCA) (2003), *Competition and Regulation in the Legal Services Market*. London: Department of Constitutional Affairs. http://www.dca.gov.uk/consult/general/oftreptconc.htm (accessed 1 December 2006).

Department of Health (DH) (1989), *Working for Patients*, Cm 555. London: HMSO.

Department of Health (DH) (1997), *The New NHS: Modern, Dependable*, Cm 3807. London: Department of Health.

Department of Health (DH) (1998), *A First Class Service: Quality in the New NHS*. London: Department of Health.

Department of Health (DH) (1999), *Making a Difference – Strengthening the Nursing, Midwifery and Health Visiting Contribution to Health and Health Care*. London: Department of Health.

Department of Health (DH) (2000a), *The NHS Plan: A Plan for Investment, a Plan for Reform*, Cm 4818-I. London: The Stationery Office.

Department of Health (DH) (2000b), *An Organisation with a Memory: Report of an Expert Group on Learning from Adverse Events in the NHS*. London: The Stationery Office.

Department of Health (DH) (2001a), *Shifting the Balance of Power within the NHS: Securing Delivery*. London: Department of Health.

Department of Health (DH) (2001b), *The Expert Patient: A New Approach to Chronic Disease Management for the 21st Century*. London: Department of Health.

Department of Health (DH) (2002a), *Delivering the NHS Plan*, Cmnd 5503. London: Stationery Office.

Department of Health (DH) (2002b), *Speech by the Right Hon Alan Milburn MP, Secretary of State, on NHS Foundation Hospitals*, 22 May. London: Department of Health.

Department of Health (DH) (2002c), *Liberating the talents – helping Primary Care Trusts and Nurses to Deliver the NHS Plan*. London: Department of Health.

Department of Health (DH) (2002d), *Shifting the Balance of Power: The Next Steps*. London: Department of Health.

Department of Health (DH) (2002e), *HR in the NHS Plan: More Staff Working Differently*. London: Department of Health.

Department of Health (DH) (2003), *Impact on Referrals and Discharge of Involving Patients and Carers in Decision-making*. London: Department of Health.

Department of Health (DH) (2004a), The *NHS Improvement Plan – Putting People at the Heart of Public Services*, Cmnd 6268. London: The Stationery Office.

Department of Health (DH) (2004b), *Choosing Health*. London: The Stationery Office.

Department of Health (DH) (2004c), *Priority Areas: First Round. Evaluation of Clinical Guidelines at the Interface*. London: Department of Health.

Department of Health (DH) (2005), *Creating a Patient-led NHS – Delivering the NHS Improvement Plan*, Gateway 4699. London: Department of Health.

Department of Health (DH) (2006a), *Hospital Episode Statistics (2006)*. London: The Stationery Office.

Department of Health (DH) (2006b), *Direction of Travel of Urgent Care*. London: The Stationery Office.

Department of Health (DH) (undated a) *The NHS Plan – Workforce*. www.doh.gov.uk/about/nhsplan/priorities/workforce.html (accessed 2 October 2002).

Department of Health (DH) (undated b) *The NHS Plan – Faster and Easier Access to Services*. www.doh.gov.uk/about/nhsplan/priorities/access.html (accessed 2 October 2002).

Department of Health (DH) (undated c) *The NHS Plan – Quality*. www.doh.gov.uk/about/nhsplan/priorities/quality.html (accessed 2 October 2002).

Department of Health and Social Security (DHSS) (1972a), *National Health Service Reorganisation: England*, Cmnd 5055. London: HMSO.

Department of Health and Social Security (DHSS) (1972b), *Management Arrangements for the Reorganised National Health Service*. London: HMSO.

Department of Health and Social Security (DHSS) (1983), *NHS Management Inquiry*. London: HMSO.

Dervitsiotis, K. (2002), The importance of conversations-for-action for effective strategic management, *Total Quality Management*, 13 (8), 1087–98.

Dickens, L. and Watkins. K. (1999), Action research: rethinking Lewin, *Management Learning*, 30 (2), 127–40.

Diefenbach, T. (2007), The managerialistic ideology of organisational change management, *Journal of Organizational Change Management*, 20 (1), 126–44.

Din, J., Newby, D. and Flapan, A. (2004), Omega 3 fatty acids and cardiovascular disease – fishing for a natural treatment, *British Medical Journal*, 328 (7430), 30–5.

DiPaola, M. and Hoy, W. (2001), Formalization, conflict, and change: constructive and destructive consequences in schools, *The International Journal of Educational Management*, 15 (5), 238–44.

Dixon, J. (2002), Foundation hospitals, *The Lancet*, 360 (9349), 1900–1.

Dobson, R. (2000), Review condemns poor leadership of Oxford cardiac services, *British Medical Journal*, 321 (7272), 1307.

Donaldson, L. (1995), Management for doctors: conflict, power, negotiation, *British Medical Journal*, 310 (6972), 104–7.

Drife, J. and Johnson, I. (1995), Management for doctors: Handling the conflicting cultures in the NHS, *British Medical Journal*, 310 (6986), 1054–6.

Drucker, P. (1989), *The New Realities*. Oxford: Heinemann Professional Publishing.

Dunphy, D. (1996), Organizational change in corporate settings, *Human Relations*, 49 (5), 541–52.

Dunphy, D. and Bryant, B. (1996), Teams: panaceas or prescriptions for improved performance? *Human Relations*, 49 (5), 677–98.

Dunphy, D., Turner, D. and Crawford, M. (1997), Organizational learning as the creation of corporate competences, *Journal of Management Development*, 16 (4), 232–44.

Eastman, W. and Bailey, J. (1994), Examining the origins of management theory: value divisions in the positive program, *Journal of Applied Behavioural Science*, 30 (3), 313–28.

Eccles, T. (1994), *Succeeding with Change: Implementing Action-driven Strategies*. London: McGraw-Hill Book Company.

Eden, C. and Huxham, C. (1996), Action research for management research, *British Journal of Management*, 7, 75–86.

Edge, K. and Laiken, M. (2002), *Changing Policy from the Inside Out: Organizational Learning in a Health-care Context*. Paper presented at the 21st Annual Conference of the Canadian Association for the Study of Adult Education (CASAE).

Edgell, S. (2006), *The Sociology of Work: Continuity and Change in Paid and Unpaid Work*. London: Sage Publications.

Edwards, N., Kornacki, M. and Silversin, J. (2002), Unhappy doctors: what are the causes and what can be done? *British Medical Journal*, 324 (7341), 835–8.

Edwards, N., Marshall, M., McLellan, A. and Abbasi, K. (2003), Doctors and managers: a problem without a solution? *British Medical Journal*, 326 (7390), 609–10.

Elden, M. and Chisholm, R. (1993), Emerging varieties of Action Research: Introduction to the Special Issue, *Human Relations*, 46 (2), 121–42.

Elliott, J. (1991), *Action Research for Educational Change*. Milton Keynes/Buckingham: Open University Press.

Elsey, H. and Lathlean, J. (2006), Using action research to stimulate organisational change within health services: experiences from two community-based studies, *Educational Action Research*, 14 (2), 171–86.

Elston, M.A. (1991), The politics of professional power: medicine in a changing health service. In: J. Gabe, M. Calnan and M. Bury (eds), *The Sociology of the Health Service*. London: Routledge. pp. 58–88.

Fagan, M. (1985), Interpersonal conflict among staff of community mental health centers, *Administration in Mental Health*, 12 (3), 192–204.

Faulkner, A. (1997), 'Strange bedfellows' in the laboratory of the NHS? An analysis of the new science of health technology assessment in the United Kingdom. In: M.A. Elston (ed.), *The Sociology of Medical Science and Technology*. Oxford: Blackwell Publishers, pp. 183–207.

Fayol, H. (revised by I. Gray) (1984), *General and Industrial Management*. New York: Institute of Electrical and Electronics Engineers Press.

Feldman, M. and Khademian, A. (2001), Principles for public management practice: from dichotomies to interdependence, *Governance: An International Journal of Policy and Administration*, 14 (3), 340–61.

Ferlie, E. and Shortell, S. (2001), Improving the Quality of Health Care in the United Kingdom and the United States: A Framework for Change, *The Milbank Quarterly*, 79 (2), 281–315.

Fisher, S., Hunter, T. and Macrosson, W. (1998), The structure of Belbin's teams, *Journal of Occupational and Organizational Psychology*, 71, 283–8.

Fisher, S., Hunter, T. and Macrosson, W. (2000), The distribution of Belbin team roles among UK managers, *Personnel Review*, 29 (2), 124–40.

Fisher, S., Macrosson, W. and Semple, J. (2001), Control and Belbin's team roles, *Personnel Review*, 30 (5), 578–88.

Fitzgerald, L., Ferlie, E., Wood, M. and Hawkins, C. (2002) Interlocking interactions, the diffusion of innovations in health care, *Human Relations*, 55 (12), 1429–49.

Fitzgerald, L., Lilley, C., Ferlie, E., Addicott, R., McGivern, G. and Buchanan, D. (2006), *Managing Change and Role Enactment in the Professionalised Organisation*. London: NCCSDO.

Fitzsimmons, P. and White, T. (1997), Medicine and management: a conflict facing general practice? *Journal of Management in Medicine*, 11 (3), 124–31.

Ford, J., Ford, L. and McNamara, R. (2002), Resistance and the background conversations of change, *Journal of Organizational Change Management*, 15 (2), 105–21.

Foucault, M. (1980), *Power/Knowledge: Selected Interviews and other Writings*. Brighton: Harvester Press.

Fox, E. and Urwick, L. (eds) (1973), *Dynamic Administration: The Collected Papers of Mary Parker Follett*, 2nd edn. New York: Hippocrene Books Inc.

Frean, A. (2000), Doctors and dentists told to 'open all hours', *The Times*, 10 March.

Freidson, E. (1970), Viewpoint: sociology and medicine: a polemic, *Sociology of Health and Illness*, 5 (2), 208–19.

Freidson, E. (1990), The centrality of professionalism to health care. *Jurimetrics Journal*, Summer, 431–45.

Frisby, W., Reid, C., Millar, S. and Hoeber, L. (2005), Putting 'participatory' into participatory forms of action research, *Journal of Sport Management*, 19, 367–86.

Galvin, K., Andrewes, C., Jackson, D., Cheesmen, S., Fudge, T., Ferris, R. and Graham, I. (1999), Investigating and implementing change within the primary health care team: issues and innovations in nursing practice, *Journal of Advanced Nursing*, 30 (1), 238–47.

Georgiades, N. and Phillimore, L. (1975), The myth of the hero-innovator and alternative strategies for organizational change. In: C. Kiernan and F. Woodford (eds), *Behaviour Modification with the Severely Mentally Retarded*. London: Associated Scientific Publishers, pp. 313–19.

Giangreco, A. and Peccei, R. (2005), The nature and antecedents of middle manager resistance to change: evidence from an Italian context, *International Journal of Human Resource Management*, 16 (10), 1812–29.

Gibson, J., Armstrong, G. and McIlveen, H. (2000), A case for reducing salt in processed foods, *Nutrition and Food Science*, 30 (4), 167–73.

Giddens, A. (1989), *Sociology*. Cambridge: Polity Press.

Gil, F., Rico, R., Alcover, C. and Barrasa, A. (2005) Change-oriented leadership, satisfaction and performance in work groups, *Journal of Managerial Psychology*, 20 (3/4), 312–28.

Gill, R. (2006), *Theory and Practice of Leadership*. London: Sage Publications.

Glencross, D. (1988), Royal Television Society lecture: '*The Future of Television*'. London: Royal Television Society, 26–7 November.

Goodlee, F. (2006), Time to leave home, *British Medical Journal*, 332, doi:10.1136/bmj.332.7544.0-f. 1 April.

Goodman, N. (2003), Foundation hospitals – we've been here before, *British Medical Journal*, 326 (7399), 1153.

Goodwin, N. (1998), Leadership in the UK NHS: where are we now? *Journal of Management in Medicine*, 12 (1), 21–32.

Goodwin, N. (2006), Healthcare system strategy and planning. In: K. Walshe and J. Smith (eds), *Healthcare Management*. Maidenhead: Open University Press, pp. 183–200.

Gorelick, C. (2005), Organizational learning vs the learning organization: a conversation with a practitioner, *The Learning Organization*, 12 (4), 383–8.

Grbich, C. (1999), *Qualitative Research in Health – An Introduction*. London: Sage Publications.

Greener, I. (2004), Talking to health managers about change: heroes, villains and simplification, *Journal of Health Organization and Management*, 18 (5), 321–35.

Greener, I. (2006), Where are the medical voices raised in protest? *British Medical Journal*, 333 (7569), 660.

Greenhalgh, T., Russell, J., Dunkley, L., Boynton, P., Lefford, F. and Chopra, N. (2006), 'We were treated like adults' – development of a pre-medicine summer school for 16 year olds from deprived socioeconomic backgrounds: action research study, *British Medical Journal*, doi:10.1136/bmj.38755.582500.55 (published 22 February). Accessed 4 November 2006.

Greenwood, A. (1997), Management/leadership: leadership for change, *Nursing Standard*, 11 (19), 22–4.

Greenwood, J. (1984), Nursing research: a position paper, *Journal of Advanced Nursing*, 9, 77–82.

Grey, C. (2005), *A Very Short, Fairly Interesting and Reasonably Cheap Book about Studying Organizations*. London: Sage Publications.

Grint, K. (1995), *Management – A Sociological Introduction*. Cambridge: Polity Press.

Grossman, L. (2006), TIME Person of the Year – You, *TIME*, 168, (27/28), 29–46.

Guardian, (2003) Tesco law reforms, *Guardian*, 26 July.

Guo, K. and Anderson, D. (2005), The new health care paradigm – roles and competencies of leaders in the service line management approach, *Leadership in Health Services*, 18 (4), xii–xx.

Hales, C. (1999), Why do managers do what they do? Reconciling evidence and theory in accounts of managerial work, *British Journal of Management*, 10, 335–50.

Hales, C. (2001), Does it matter what managers do? *Business Strategy Review*, 12 (2), 50–8.

Hall, J.E. (2006), Professionalizing action research – a meaningful strategy for modernizing services? *Journal of Nursing Management*, 14, 195–200.

Hammersley, M. (2004), Action research: a contradiction in terms? *Oxford Review of Education*, 30 (2), 165–81.

Handy, C. (1993), *Understanding Organisations*, 4th edn. London: Penguin.

Harding, N. (1998), The social construction of management. In: A. Symmonds and A. Kelly (eds), *The Social Construction of Community Care*. Basingstoke: Macmillan.

Harrison, S. and Ahmed, W. (2000) Medical autonomy and the UK state 1975–2025, *Sociology*, 34 (1), 129–46.

Harrison, S. and Lim, J. (2003), The frontier of control: doctors and managers in the NHS, 1966–1997, *Clinical Governance*, 8 (1), 13–18.

Hart, E. (1996), Action research as a professionalizing strategy: issues and dilemmas, *Journal of Advanced Nursing*, 23 (3), 454–61.

Hart, E. and Bond, M. (1995), *Action Research for Health and Social Care – A Guide to Practice*. Buckingham: Open University Press.

Hartley, J. and Hinkson, B. (2003), *Leadership Development: A Systematic Review of the Literature: A Report for the NHS leadership Centre*. Coventry: Warwick Institute of Governance and Public Management, Warwick Business School, University of Warwick.

Hartley, J., Bennington, J. and Binns, P. (1997), Researching the roles of internal-change agents in the management of organizational change, *British Journal of Management*, 8, 61–73.

Harvey-Jones, J. (1990), Shropshire District Health Authority, in *Trouble Shooter*. London: BBC Books, 127–49.

Haug, M. (1988), A re-examination of the hypothesis of physician deprofessionalization, *The Milbank Quarterly*, 66, Supp. 2, 48–58.

Havard, J. (2004), Letter: nature of NHS funding slows change, *The Times*, 10 May.

Hawkes, S. (2008), Feeling unwell? Just pop down to the supermarket to see the GP, *The Times*, 22 February.

Healthcare Commission (2006), *State of Healthcare 2006*. London: Commission for Healthcare Audit and Inspection.

Healthcare Commission (2007), *Spotlight on Complaints*. London: Commission for Healthcare Audit and Inspection.

Hedley, A., Fennell, S., Wall, D. and Cullen, R. (2003), People will support what they help to create: clinical governance large group work, *Clinical Governance: An International Journal*, 8 (2), 174–9.

Helman, C. (1990), *Culture, Health and Illness*, 2nd edn. London: Wright.

Hendry, C. (1996), Understanding and creating whole organizational change through learning theory, *Human Relations*, 49 (5), 621–41.

Hewison, A. (2001), The modern matron: reborn or recycled, *Journal of Nursing Management*, 9, 187–9.

Hewison, A. and Griffiths, M. (2004), Leadership development in health care: a word of caution, *Journal of Health Organization and Management*, 18 (6), 464–73.

Hilgard, E. and Atkinson, R. (1967), *Introduction to Psychology*, 4th edn. New York: Harcourt, Brace.

Hjul, J. (2006), Comment: let GPs go private to do their job well, *Sunday Times Scotland*, 17 December.

Hoag, B., Ritschard, H. and Cooper, G. (2002), Obstacles to effective organizational change: the underlying reasons, *Leadership & Organization Development Journal*, 23 (1), 6–15.

Hodgkin, P. (1996), Medicine, postmodernism, and the end of certainty, *British Medical Journal*, 313 (7072), 1568–9.

Hofstede, G. (1998), Attitudes, values, and organizational culture: Disentangling the concepts, *Organization Studies*, 19 (3), 477–92.

Holland, C. (1993), An ethnographic study of nursing culture as an exploration for determining the existence of a system of ritual, *Journal of Advanced Nursing*, 18, 1461–70.

Holter, I.G. and Schwartz-Barcott, D. (1993), Action research: what is it? How has it been used and how can it be used in nursing? *Journal of Advanced Nursing*, 18, 298–304.

Hope, K. and Waterman, H. (2003). Praiseworthy pragmatism? Validity and action research, *Journal of Advanced Nursing*, 44 (20), 120–7.

Hounshell, D. (1984), *The American System of Mass Production 1800–1932: The Development of Manufacturing Technology in the United States*. Baltimore: Johns Hopkins University Press.

House of Commons Health Committee (2004), *Obesity: Third Report of Session 2003/4*, HC 23-I. London: House of Commons/The Stationery Office.

Howe, D. (1994), Modernity, postmodernity and social work, *British Journal of Social Work*, 24, 513–32.

Howkins, E. and Thornton, C. (2002), *Managing and Leading Innovation in Health Care*. London: Bailliere Tindall.

Huczynski, A. and Buchanan, D. (2001), *Organisational Behaviour: An Introductory Text*, 4th edn. London: Prentice Hall.

Hunt, J. (1992), *Managing People at Work: A Manager's Guide to Behaviour in Organizations*, 3rd edn. London: The McGraw-Hill Companies.

Hunter, D. (1991), Managing medicine: a response to the crisis, *Social Science and Medicine*, 32 (4), 441–9.

Hunter, D. (1992), Doctors as managers: poachers turned gamekeepers? *Social Science and Medicine*, 35 (4), 557–66.

Hunter, D. (1994), From tribalism to corporatism: the managerial challenge to medical dominance. In: J. Gabe, D. Kellerher and G. Williams (eds), *Challenging Medicine*. London: Routledge. pp. 1–22.

Hyde, P. and Davies, H.T.O. (2004) Service design, culture and performance: collusion and co-production in health care, *Human Relations*, 57 (11), 1407–26.

Hyett, E. (2003), What blocks health visitors from taking on a leadership role? *Journal of Nursing Management*, 11, 229–33.

Illich, I. (1977), *Limits to Medicine, Medical Nemesis: The Expropriation of Health.* Harmondsworth: Penguin Books.

Jarrett, M. (2003), The seven myths of change management, *Business Strategy Review*, 14 (4), 22–9.

Jehn, K. (1995), A multimethod examination of the benefits and detriments of intra-group conflict, *Administrative Science Quarterly*, 40 (2), 256–82.

Jessop, B. (1994), The transition to post-Fordism and the Schumpeterian workfare state. In: R. Burrows and B. Loader (eds), *Towards a Post-Fordist Welfare State?* London: Routledge, pp.13–37.

Johnson, G. (1993), Processes of managing strategic change. In: C. Mabey and B. Mayon-White (eds), *Managing Change*, 2nd edn. London: Paul Chapman Publishing, pp. 59–84.

Johnson, G. and Scholes, K. (1989), *Exploring Corporate Strategy: Texts and Cases.* New York: Prentice Hall.

Johnson, J. (1998), Embracing change: a leadership model for the learning organisation, *International Journal of Training and Development*, 2 (2), 141–50.

Jooste, K. (2004), Leadership: a new perspective, *Journal of Nursing Management*, 12, 217–23.

Juhl, H., Eskildsen, J. and Kristensen, K. (2004), Conflict or congruence? The case of a Danish hospital, *International Journal of Quality & Reliability Management*, 21 (7), 747–62.

Kakabadse, A. (2000), From individual to team to cadre: tracking leadership for the third millennium, *Strategic Change*, 9, 5–16.

Kegan, R. and Lahey, L.L. (2001), The real reason people won't change, *Harvard Business Review*, 79 (10), 85–92.

Keller, R. (1995), 'Transformational leaders make a difference, *Research Technology Management*, 38 (3), 41–4.

Kelleher, D., Gabe, J. and Williams, G. (1994), Understanding medical dominance in the modern world. In: J. Gabe, D. Kelleher and G. Williams (eds), *Challenging Medicine.* London: Routledge, pp. xi–xxix.

Kelly, D., Simpson, S. and Brown, P. (2002), An action research project to evaluate the clinical practice facilitator role for junior nurses in an acute hospital setting, *Journal of Clinical Nursing*, 11, 90–8.

Kennedy, I. (2001), *Learning from Bristol: The Report of the Public Inquiry into Children's Heart Surgery at the Bristol Royal Infirmary 1984–1995*, Cm 5207(I). London: The Stationery Office.

Kermode, S. and Brown, C. (1996), The postmodernist hoax and its effects on nursing, *International Journal of Nursing Studies*, 33 (4), 375–84.

King's Fund (2005), *Putting Health in Local Hands: Early Experiences of Homerton University Hospital NHS Foundation Trust.* London: King's Fund Publications.

Kinnunen, J. (1990), The importance of organisational culture on development activities in a primary health care organization, *International Journal of Health Planning and Management*, 5, 65–71.

Kirkham, M. (1999), The culture of midwifery in the National Health Service in England, *Journal of Advanced Nursing*, 30 (3), 732–9.

Klein, R. (1999), Grating expectations, *The Guardian*, 20 October.

Knightbridge, S., King, R. and Rolfe, T. (2006), Using participatory action research in a community-based initiative addressing mental health needs, *Australian and New Zealand Journal of Psychiatry*, 40 (40), 325–32.

Koeck, C. (1998), Time for organisational development in healthcare organizations, *British Medical Journal*, 317 (7168), 1267–8.

Kolb, D. (1984), *Experiential Learning*, Englewood Cliffs, NJ: Prentice Hall.

Kotter, J.P. (1990), *A Force for Change: How Leadership Differs from Management*. New York: Free Press.

Krantz, J. (1999), Comment on 'Challenging resistance to change', *Journal of Applied Behavioral Science*, 35 (1), 42–4.

Kumar, K. and Thibodeaux, M. (1990), Organizational politics and planned organizational change, *Group and Organizational Studies*, 15 (4), 357–65.

Lamb, M. and Cox, M. (1999), Implementing change in the National Health Service, *Journal of Management in Medicine*, 13 (5), 288–97.

Laming, Lord (2003), *The Victoria Climbié Inquiry: Report of an Inquiry*, CM 5730. London: Secretary of State for Health and the Secretary of State for the Home Department.

Lathlean, J. and le May, A. (2002), Communities of practice: an opportunity for interagency working, *Journal of Clinical Nursing*, 11, 394–8.

Lean, M., Gruer, L., Alberti, G. and Satter, N. (2006), Obesity – can we turn the tide? *British Medical Journal*, 333 (7581), 1261–4.

Learmonth, M. (2005), Doing things with words: The case of 'management' and 'administration', *Public Administration*, 83 (3), 617–37.

Le Grand, J., Mays, N. and Mulligan, J.-A. (1998), *Learning from the NHS Internal Market – A Review of the Evidence*. London: King's Fund.

Leighton, K. (2005), Action research: the revision of services at one mental health rehabilitation unit in the north of England, *Journal of Psychiatric and Mental Health Nursing*, 12, 372–9.

Lemak, D. (2004), Leading students through the management theory jungle by following the path of the seminal theorists – A paradigmatic approach, *Management Decisions*, 42 (10), 1309–25.

Lewin, K. (1942/1997), Field theory and learning, *in Resolving Social Conflicts & Field Theory in Social Science*. Washington, DC: American Psychological Association, pp. 212–30.

Lewin, K. (1946), Action research and minority problems, *Journal of Social Issues*, 2, 34–46.

Lewin, K. (1946/1997), Behaviour and development as a function of the total situation, in *Resolving Social Conflicts & Field Theory in Social Science*. Washington, DC: American Psychological Association, 337–81.

Lewin, K. (1947/1997), Frontiers in group dynamics, in *Resolving Social Conflicts & Field Theory in Social Science*. Washington, DC: American Psychological Association, pp. 301–36.

Lilford, R., Warren, R. and Braunholtz, D. (2003), Action research: a way of researching or a way of managing? *Journal of Health Services Research and Policy*, 8 (2), 100–4.

Lindsey, E. and McGuiness, L. (1998), Significant elements of community involvement in participatory action research: evidence from a community project, *Journal of Advanced Nursing*, 28 (5), 1106–14.

Lindsey, E., Shields, L. and Stajduhar, K. (1999), Creating effective nursing partnerships: relating community development to participatory action research, *Journal of Advanced Nursing*, 29 (5), 1238–45.

Lippitt, R., Watson, J. and Westley, B. (1958), *The Dynamics of Planned Change*. New York: Harcourt, Brace.

Lipshitz, R. and Popper, M. (2000), Organizational learning in a hospital, *The Journal of Applied Organizational Behavioral Science*, 36 (3), 345–61.

Lister, S. (2005), GPs must open round the clock, *The Times*, 11 November.

Livesey, H. and Challender, S. (2002), Supporting organizational learning: a comparative approach to evaluation in action research, *Journal of Nursing Management*, 10, 167–76.

Lyotard, F. (1984), *The Postmodern Condition: A Report on Knowledge*. Manchester: Manchester University Press.

Mabin, V., Forgeson, S. and Green, L. (2001), Harnessing resistance: using the theory of constraints to assist change management, *Journal of European Industrial Training*, 25, (2/3/4), 168–91.

Macaulay, A., Commanda, L., Freeman, W., Gibson, N., McCabe, M., Robbins, C. and Twohig, P. (1999), Participatory research maximises community and lay involvement, *British Medical Journal*, 319 (7212), 774–8.

Macfarlane, F., Gantley, M. and Murray, E. (2002), The CeMENT project: a case study in change management, *Medical Teacher*, 24 (3), 320–6.

Machiavelli, N. (1532/1979), The Prince. In: P. Bondanella and M. Musa (eds), *The Portable Machiavelli*. London: Penguin. pp. 77–166.

Magee, J., Pritchard, E., Fitzgerald, K., Dunstan, F. and Howard, A. (1999), Antibiotic prescribing and antibiotic resistance in community practice: retrospective study, 1996–8, *British Medical Journal*, 319 (7219), 1239–40.

Manley, K. (2000), Organisational culture and consultant nurse outcomes: Part 1: organisational culture, *Nursing Standard*, 14 (36), 34–8.

Mannion, R., Davies, H. and Marshall, M. (2005), *Cultures for Performance in Health Care*. Maidenhead: Open University Press.

Marincowitz, G.J.O. (2003), How to use participatory action research in primary care, *Family Practice*, 20 (5), 595–600.

Marsh, I. (ed.) (2000), *Sociology: Making Sense of Society*, 2nd edn. Harlow: Prentice Hall.

Marshall, M., Noble, J., Davies, H., Waterman, H., Walshe, K., Sheaff, R. and Elwyn, G. (2006), Development of an information source for patients and the public about general practice services: an action research study, *Health Expectation*, 9, 265–74.

Martins, E. and Terblanche, F. (2003), Building organizational culture that stimulates creativity and innovation, *European Journal of Innovation Management*, 6 (1), 64–74.

Massey, L. and Williams, S. (2006), Implementing change: the perspective of NHS change agents, *Leadership and Organization Development Journal*, 27 (8), 667–81.

May, T. (2001), *Social Research: Issues, Methods and Process*, 3rd edn. Buckingham: Open University Press.

McAdam, R. (2005), A multi-level theory of innovation implementation: Normative evaluation, legitimization and conflict, *European Journal of Innovation Management*, 8 (3), 373–88.

McElhaney, R. (1996), Conflict management in nursing administration, *Nursing Management*, 27 (3), 49–50.

McHugh, M., Johnson, K. and McClelland, D. (2007), HRM and the management of clinicians within the NHS, *International Journal of Public Sector Management*, 20 (4), 314–24.

McKenna, H., Keeney, S. and Bradley, M. (2004), Nurse leadership within primary care: the perceptions of community nurses, GPs, policy makers and members of the public, *Journal of Nursing Management*, 12, 69–76.

McLarney, C. and Rhyno, S. (1999), Mary Parker Follett: visionary leadership and strategic management, *Women in Management Review*, 14 (7), 292–302.

McMurray, A. and Williams, L. (2004), Factors impacting on nurse managers' ability to be innovative in a decentralized management structure, *Journal of Nursing Management*, 12, 348–53.

McWilliam, C. and Ward-Griffin, C. (2006), Implementing organizational change in health and social services, *Journal of Organizational Change Management*, 19 (2), 119–35.

Medina, F., Munduate, L., Dorado, M., Martínez, I. and Guerra, J. (2005), Types of intra-group conflict and affective reactions, *Journal of Managerial Psychology*, 20 (3/4), 219–30.

Meldrum, H. (2006), General practice under pressure, *British Medical Journal*, 332 (7532), 46–7.

Merali, F. (2003), NHS managers' views of their culture and their public image: implications for NHS reforms, *The International Journal of Public Sector Management*, 16 (7), 549–63.

Meyer, J. (1995), Action research: stages in the process: a personal account, *Nurse Researcher*, 2 (3), 24–37.

Meyer, J. (2000), Using qualitative methods in health related action research, *British Medical Journal*, 320 (7228), 178–81.

Michie, S. and West, M. (2004), Managing people and performance: an evidence based framework applied to health service organizations. *International Journal of Management Reviews*, 5/6 (2), 91–111.

Mill, J.S. (1910), *Utilitarianism, Liberty and Representative Government*. London: Dent.

Miller, D. (2000), *Leading an Empowered Organization. Creative Healthcare Management*, Leeds: CDNPP, University of Leeds.

Millward, L. and Bryan, K. (2005), Clinical leadership in health care: a position statement, *Leadership in Health Services*, 18(2), xiii–xxv.

Mintzberg, H. (1994), *The Rise and Fall of Strategic Planning*. New Jersey: Prentice Hall.

Mitchell, E., Conlon, A.-M., Armstrong, M. and Ryan, A. (2005), Towards rehabilitative handling in caring for patients following stroke: a participatory action research project, *Journal of Clinical Nursing*, 14 (3a), 3–12.

Mohan, J. (1995), Post-Fordism and welfare: an analysis of change in the British health sector, *Environment and Planning*, 27, 1555–76.

Mohan, J. (2003), The past and future of the NHS: new Labour and foundation hospitals, *History and Policy*, www.historyandpolicy.org/archive/policy-paper-14.html (accessed 23 November 2006).

Morgan, G. (1993) Organizations as political systems. In: C. Mabey and B. Mayon-White (eds), *Managing Change*, 2nd edn. London: Paul Chapman Publishing, pp. 212–17.

Morgan, G. (1998), *Images of Organizations: The Executive Edition*. Thousand Oaks, CA: Sage Publications.

Morrison, B. and Lilford, R. (2001), How can action research apply to health services?, *Qualitative Health Research*, 11 (4), 436–49.

Mrayyan, M. (2004), Nurses' autonomy: influence of nurse managers' actions, *Journal of Advanced Nursing*, 45 (3), 326–36.

Muir Gray, J.A. (1999), Postmodern medicine, *The Lancet*, 354 (9189), 1550–3.

Mullally, S. (2003) Keynote Address, at Chief Nursing Officers Conference: London. http://www.dh.gov.uk/en/News/Speeches/Speecheslist/DH_4066718 (accessed 1 November 2007).

Murphy, L. (2005), Transformational leadership: a cascading chain reaction, *Journal of Nursing Management*, 13, 128–36.

Nadler, D. (1993), Concepts for the management of organizational change. In: C. Mabey and B. Mayon-White (eds), *Managing Change*, 2nd edn. London: Paul Chapman Publishing, pp. 85–98.

National Audit Office, (2006), *The Provision of Out-of-Hours Care in England*. London: The Stationery Office.

National Health Service (NHS) (2005), *A Short Guide to NHS Foundation Trusts*. Gateway 5591. London: Department of Health.

National Health Service Executive (NHSE) (2000), *Report of the External Review into Oxford Cardiac Services*, London: South East Regional Office/NHSE.

Naylor, D. (2006), Leadership in academic medicine: reflections from administrative exile. *The Lilley Lecture 2006*. London: Royal College of Physicians, http://rcplondon.ac.uk/event/details.aspx?e=301 Video: https://admin.emea.acrobat.com/_a45839050/p39801080/(accessed 1 June 2007).

Newbold, D. (2005), Foundation Trusts: economics in the 'post-modern hospital', *Journal of Nursing Management*, 13, 439–47.

NHS Modernisation Board, (2002), *The NHS Plan – A Progress Report. Annual Report 2000–2001*. London: NHS Modernisation Board.

NICE, (2005), *A Guide to NICE*, London: National Institute for Health and Clinical Excellence.

Nichols, R. (1997), Action research in health care: the Collaborative Action Research Network Health Care Group, *Educational Action Research*, 5 (2), 185–92.

Nicholson, N. (1993), Organizational change. In C. Mabey and B. Mayon-White (eds), *Managing Change*, 2nd edn. London: Paul Chapman Publishing, pp. 207–11.

Northouse, P. (2004) *Leadership: Theory and Practice*, 3rd edn. Thousand Oaks: Sage Publications.

NZRU (2003), http://www.allblacks.com/index.cfm?layout=haka (accessed 9 August 2007).

O'Brien, R. (1998/2001), An overview of the methodological approach of action research. In: Roberto Richardson (ed.), *Theory and Practice of Action Research*. João Pessoa, Brazil: Universidade Federal da Paraíba. http://www.web.ca/~robrien/papers/arfinal.html (accessed 20 January 2002).

Office for National Statistics (ONS) (2005), *The Labour Force Survey*, London: Statistical Office.

Office for National Statistics (ONS) (2006a), *Social Trends 36*. Basingstoke: Palgrave.

Office for National Statistics (ONS) (2006b), *Hospital and Family Health Services (England and Wales)*. http://www.statistics.gov.uk/STATBASE/Expodata/Spreadsheets/D3979.xls (accessed 15 December 2006).

Oldcorn, R. (1996), *Management*, 3rd edn. Basingstoke: Macmillan Business.

Olsen, S. and Neale, G. (2005), Clinical leadership in the provision of hospital care, *British Medical Journal*, 330 (7502), 1219–20, 28 May.

O'Mathúna, D.P. (2004), The future of nursing: postmodernism and nursing: after the honeymoon, *Journal of Christian Nursing Education*, 21 (3), 4–11.

Oreg, S. (2006), Personality, context and resistance to organizational change, *European Journal of Work and Organizational Psychology*, 15 (1), 73–101.

Orgland, M. (1997), *Initiating, Managing and Sustaining Strategic Change – Learning from the Best*. Basingstoke: Macmillan Business.

Orlikowski, W.J. (1996), Improvising organizational transformations over time: a situated change perspective, *Information Systems Research*, 7 (1), 63–92.

Osborne, H. (2006), Firms offered help shrinking carbon footprints, *Guardian*, 21 November.

O'Toole, J. (1995), *Leading Change: Overcoming the Ideology of Comfort and the Tyranny of Custom*. San Francisco: Jossey-Bass.

Outhwaite, S. (2003), The importance of leadership in the development of an integrated team, *Journal of Nursing Management*, 11, 371–6.

Pacanowsky, M.E. and O'Donnell-Trujillo, N. (1982), Communication and organizational cultures, *Western Journal of Speech Communication*, 46 (2), 115–30.

Padaki, V. (2002), Making the organization learn: demystification and management action, *Development in Practice*, 12 (3 & 4), 321–37.

Pardo del Val, M. and Martinez Fuentes, C. (2003), Resitance to change: a literature review and empirical study, *Management Decision*, 41 (2), 148–55.

Parker, L. and Ritson, P. (2005), Fads, stereotypes and management gurus: Fayol and Follett today, *Management Decision*, 43 (10), 1335–57.

Parkin, P. (1997), Managing Change in the Community. In: S. Burley and E.E. Mitchell (eds), *Contemporary Community Nursing*. London: Edward Arnold, pp. 132–54.

Parkin, P. (1998), An approach to management for community health professionals, *British Journal of Community Nursing*, 3 (8), 374–81.

Parkin, P. (1999a), Managing change in the community 1: the case of PCGs, *British Journal of Community Nursing*, 4 (1), 19–27.

Parkin, P. (1999b), Managing change in the community 2: partnership in PCGs, *British Journal of Community Nursing*, 4 (4), 188–95.

Parkin, P. (1999c), Managing change in the community 3: conflict in PCGs, *British Journal of Community Nursing*, 4 (6), 275–82.

Passos, A. and Caetano, A. (2005), Exploring the effects of intragroup conflict and past performance feedback on team effectiveness, *Journal of Managerial Psychology*, 20 (3/4), 231–44.

Paton, R.A. and McCalman, J. (2000), *Change Management: A Guide to Effective Implementation*, 2nd edn. London: Sage Publications.

Peck, E. (2006), Leadership and its development in healthcare. In: K. Walshe and J. Smith (eds), *Healthcare Management*. Maidenhead: Open University Press, pp. 323–41.

Pension Service, The (2008), *Pensions – the Basics*, London: The Pensions Service, Department of Work and Pensions.

Perren, L. and Megginson, D. (1996), Resistance to change as a positive force: its dynamics and issues for management development, *Career Development International*, 1 (4), 24–8.

Peters, T. (1978), Symbols, patterns and settings, *Organizational Dynamics*, 7 (2), 3–23.

Pettigrew, A. (1979), On studying organizational cultures, *Administrative Science Quarterly*, 24, 570–81.

Pettigrew, A., Ferlie, E. and McKee, L. (1992), *Shaping Strategic Change: Making Change in Large Organizations: The Case of the National Health Service*, London: Sage.

Pickersgill, T. (2001), The European working time directive for doctors in training, *British Medical Journal*, 323 (7339), 1266.

Piderit, S. (2000), Rethinking resistance and recognising ambivalence: a multidimensional view of attitudes toward an original change, *Academy of Management Review*, 25 (4), 783–94.

Plsek, P. and Greenhalgh, T. (2001), The challenge of complexity in health care, *British Medical Journal*, 323 (7313), 625–8.

Plsek, P and Wilson, T. (2001), Complexity, leadership, and management in healthcare organisations, *British Medical Journal*, 323 (7315), 746–9.

Pollitt, C. (1993), *Managerialism and the Public Services: Cuts or Culture Change in the 1990s*, 2nd edn. Oxford: Blackwell.

Pollock, A. (2005), *NHS plc – The Privatization of our Health Care*. London: Verso.

Potter, C., Morgan, P. and Thompson, A. (1994), Continuous quality improvement in an acute hospital: A report of an action research project in three hospital departments. *International Journal of Health Care Quality Assurance*, 7 (1), 4–29.

Preston, D., Smith, A., Buchanan, D. and Jordan, S. (1996), Symbols of the NHS – understanding the culture and communication processes of a general hospital, *Management Learning*, 27 (3), 343–57.

Procter, S., Currie, G. and Orme, H. (1999), The empowerment of middle managers in a community trust: structure, responsibility and culture, *Personnel Review*, 28 (3), 242–57.

Pruijt, H. (2000), Repainting, modifying, smashing Taylorism, *Journal of Organizational Change*, 13 (5), 439–51.

Pryjmachuk, S. (1996), Pragmatism and change: some implications for nurses, nurse managers and nursing, *Journal of Nursing Management*, 4, 201–5.

Pyrch, T. (2007), Participatory action research and the culture of fear, *Action Research*, 5 (2), 199–216.

Quoss, B., Cooney, M. and Longhurst, T. (2000), Academics and advocates: using participatory action research to influence welfare policy, *The Journal of Consumer Affairs*, 34 (1), 47–61.

Rahim, M.A. (1985), A strategy for managing conflict in complex organizations, *Human Relations*, 38 (1), 81–9.

Rahim, M. and Bonoma, T. (1979), Managing organizational conflict: a model for diagnosis and intervention, *Psychological Reports*, 44, 1323–44.

Raithatha, N. (1997), Medicine, postmodernism, and the end of certainty, *British Medical Journal*, 314 (7086), 1044.

Reason, P. (2001), Learning and change through action research. In: J. Henry (ed.), *Creative Management*. London: Sage Publications, pp. 182–94.

Reay, B. (2004), Letter: NHS Management, *The Times*, 2 January.

Reay, T., Golden-Biddle, K. and Germann, K. (2003), Challenges and leadership strategies for managers of nurse practitioners, *Journal of Nursing Management*, 11, 396–403.

Reed, J. (2005), Using action research in nursing practice with older people: democratizing knowledge, *Journal of Clinical Nursing*, 14, 594–600.

Reedy, P. and Learmonth, M. (2000), Nursing managers, transformed or deformed? A case study in the ideology of competency, *Journal of Management in Medicine*, 14 (3/4), 153–65.

Reid, G., Kneafsey, R., Long, A., Hulme, C. and Wright, H. (2007), Change and transformation: the impact of an action research evaluation on the development of a new service, *Learning in Health and Social Care*, 6 (2), 61–71.

Reform, (2004) *Bulletin Archive 31 March 2004*. London: Reform. www.reform.co.uk/website/pressroom/bulletinarchive.aspx?o=69 (accessed 6 December 2006).

Rhydderch, M., Elwyn, G., Marshall, M. and Grol, R. (2004), Organisational change theory and the use of indicators in general practice, *Quality and Safety in Health Care*, 13, 213–17.

Rogers, C. (1983), *Freedom to Learn for the 80's*. London: Charles Merrill Publishing.

Rolfe, G. (1996), Going to extremes: action research, grounded practice and the theory–practice gap in nursing, *Journal of Advanced Nursing*, 24 (6), 1315–20.

Rolfe, G. (2001), Postmodernism for healthcare workers in 13 easy steps, *Nurse Education Today*, 21, 38–47.

Rolfe, G. (2006), Judgements without rules: towards a postmodern ironist concept of research validity, *Nursing Inquiry*, 13 (1), 7–15.

Rose, A. (2005), Letter: doctors' guidelines from primary care trusts, *The Times*, 21 June.

Rowden, R.W. (2001), The learning organization and strategic change, *S.A.M. Advanced Management Journal*, 66 (3), 11–24.

Royal Pharmaceutical Society (2000), *Team-working in Primary Healthcare*. London: Royal Pharmaceutical Society/British Medical Association.

Rushmer, R., Lough, M., Wilkenson, J. and Davies, H.T.O. (2004a), Introducing the Learning Practice – III. Leadership, empowerment, protected time and reflective practice as core contextual conditions, *Journal of Evaluation in Clinical Practice*, 10 (3), 399–405.

Rushmer, R., Lough, M., Wilkenson, J. and Davies, H.T.O. (2004b), Introducing the Learning Practice – I. The characteristics of learning organizations in primary care, *Journal of Evaluation in Clinical Practice*, 10 (3), 375–86.

Rushmer, R., Kelly, D., Lough, M., Wilkenson, J. and Davies, H.T.O. (2004c), Introducing the Learning Practice – II. Becoming a Learning Practice. *Journal of Evaluation in Clinical Practice*, 10 (3), 387–98.

Russell, B. (1950), Philosophy and politics, in *Unpopular Essays*. London: Allen and Unwin.

Saka, A. (2003), Internal change agents' views of the management of change problem, *Journal of Organizational Change Management*, 16 (5), 480–96.

Salauroo, M. and Burnes, B. (1998), The impact of a market system on the public sector: a study of organizational change in the NHS, *International Journal of Public Sector Management*, 11 (6), 451–67.

Salimath, M. and Lemak, D. (2005), Mary P. Follett: translating philosophy into a paradigm of lifelong learning, *Management Decision*, 42 (10), 1284–96.

Salvage, J. and Smith, R. (2000), Doctors and nurses: doing it differently, *British Medical Journal*, 320 (7241), 1019–20.

Sambrook, S. (2006), Management development in the NHS: nurses and managers, discourses and identities, *Journal of European Industrial Training*, 30 (1), 48–64.

Sandars, J. and Waterman, H. (2005), Using action research to improve and understand professional practice, *Work Based Learning in Primary Care*, 3, 294–305.

Savage, J. (2000), The culture of culture in National Health Service policy implementation, *Nursing Inquiry*, 7, 230–8.

Scambler, G. (2002), *Health and Social Change*. Buckingham: Open University Press.

Schein, E. (1985), *Organisational Culture and Leadership*. San Francisco: Jossey-Bass.

Schein, E. (2004), *Organisational Culture and Leadership*, 3rd edn. San Francisco: Jossey-Bass.

Schwartz, C. (Chief Editor), (1988), *Chambers Concise Dictionary*. Edinburgh: Chambers Harrap.

Scott, T., Mannion, R., Davies, H.T.O. and Marshall, M. (2003), Implementing culture change in health care: theory and practice, *International Journal for Quality in Health Care*, 15 (2), 111–18.

Scrivens, E. (1988), Doctors and managers: never the twain shall meet, *British Medical Journal*, 296 (6639), 1754–5.

Seidman, S. (1994), *Contested Knowledge: Social Theory in the Postmodern Era*. Oxford: Blackwell.

Seymour, F. and Davies, E. (2002), Using action research to facilitate change in child protection services, *Journal of Community Psychology*, 30 (5), 585–90.

Shani, A. and Eberhardt, B. (1987), Parallel organization in a health care institution: An exploratory action research study, *Group and Organizational Studies*, 12 (2), 147–73.

Shannon, C. (2003), Freedoms of Foundation Hospitals don't go far enough, *British Medical Journal*, 327 (7422), 1008.

Shannon, C. (2007), MTAS: where are we now? *British Medical Journal*, 334 (7598) 824–5.

Sheaff, M. (2005), *Sociology & Health Care*, Maidenhead: Open University Press.

Simons, J. (2002), An action research study exploring how education may enhance pain management in children, *Nurse Education Today*, 22, 108–17.

Sims Jr., H.P. and Lorenzi, P. (1992), *The New Leadership Paradigm: Social Learning and Cognition in Organizations*. Newbury Park, CA: Sage Publications.

Singh, R. (2005), Sex disease tests at Boots in NHS deal, *Evening Standard*, 7 February.

Skjørshammer, M. (2001), Co-operation and conflict in a hospital: interprofessional differences in perception and management of conflicts, *Journal of Interprofessional Care*, 15 (1), 7–18.

Smallwood, S. and Chamberlain, J. (2005), Replacement fertility: what has it been and what does it mean? *Population Trends*, 119, 16–27.

Smart, B. (1993), *Postmodernity*. London: Routledge.

Smith, I. and Boyns, T. (2005) British management theory and practice: the impact of Fayol, *Management Decision*, 43 (10), 1317–34.

Smith, R. (2002), Oh NHS, thou art sick, *British Medical Journal*, 324 (7330), 127–8.

Smith, R. (2003a), Changing the 'leadership' of the NHS, *British Medical Journal*, 326, doi:10.1136/bmj.326.7403.0-g. 21 June.

Smith, R. (2003b), What doctors and managers can learn from each other. *British Medical Journal*, 326 (7390), 610–11.

Spitzer, A. (1998), Nursing in the health care system of the post-modern world: crossroads, paradoxes and complexity, *Journal of Advanced Nursing*, 28 (1), 164–71.

Staniforth, D. and West, M. (1995), Leading and managing teams, *Team Performance Management: An International Journal*, 1 (2), 28–33.

Stewart, J. and O'Donnell, M. (2007), Implementing change in a public agency – leadership, learning and organizational resilience, *International Journal of Public Sector Management*, 20 (3), 239–51.

Stringer, E. (1996), *Action Research: A Handbook for Practitioners*. Thousand Oaks, CA: Sage Publications.

Stoney, C. (2001), Strategic management or Taylorism? A case study into change within a UK local authority, *The International Journal of Public Sector Management*, 14 (1), 27–42.

Stordeur, S., D'hoore, W. and Vandenberghe, C. (2001), Leadership, organizational stress, and emotional exhaustion among hospital nursing staff, *Journal of Advanced Nursing*, 35 (4), 533–42.

Sunday Times, (2003), Editorial: hospitals of hope, *The Sunday Times*, 4 May.

Taylor, B. (2001), Identifying and transforming dysfunctional nurse–nurse relationships through reflective practice and action research, *International Journal of Nursing Practice*, 7, 406–13.

Taylor, F.W. (1911/1967), *The Principles of Scientific Management*. New York: W.W. Norton and Company.

Taylor, R., Braveman, B. and Hammel, J. (2004), Developing and evaluating community-based services through participatory action research: Two case examples, *The American Journal of Occupational Therapy*, 58, 73–82.

Thomas, K. and Kilmann, R. (1974), *Thomas-Kilmann Conflict Mode Instrument*. Tuxedo, NY: XICOM Inc.

Thomas, P., McDonnell, J., McCulloch, J., While, A., Bosenquet, N. and Ferlie, E. (2005), Increasing capacity for innovation in bureaucratic organizations: a whole system participatory action research project, *Annals of Family Medicine*, 3 (4), 312–17.

Thompson, D. (1987), Coalitions and conflict in the National Health Service: some implications for general management, *Sociology of Health and Illness*, 9 (2), 127–53.

Thorne, M.L. (1997), Myth management in the NHS, *Journal of Management in Medicine*, 11 (3), 168–80.

Times, The (2000), Editorial: health warning: the NHS Plan requires more than a short-term strategy, *The Times*, 20 November.

Timpson, J. (1998), The NHS as a learning organization: aspirations beyond the rainbow? *Journal of Nursing Management*, 6, 261–74.

Tolliday, H. (1976), Clinical autonomy. In E. Jaques, (ed.), *Health Services: Their Nature and Organization and the Role of Patients, Doctors, Nurses and the Complementary Professions*. London: Heineman, pp. 32–52.

Treasure, T. (2001), Redefining leadership in health care, *British Medical Journal*, 323, 1263–4.

Trofino, J. (1995), Transformational leadership in health care, *Nursing Management*, 26 (8), 42–7.

Tuckett, D., Boulton, M., Olson, C. and Williams, A. (1985), *Meetings Between Experts*. London: Tavistock.

Valentine, P. (2001), A gender perspective on conflict management strategies of nurses, *Journal of Nursing Scholarship*, 33 (1), 69–74.

Van Wart, M. (2003), Public-sector leadership theory: an assessment, *Public Administration Review*, 63 (2), 214–28.

Waddell, D. and Sohal, A. (1998), Resistance: a constructive tool for change, *Management Decision*, 36 (8), 543–8.

Walby, S. and Greenwell, J. with MacKay, L. and Soothill, K. (1994), *Medicine and Nursing: Professions in a Changing Health Service*. London: Sage Publications.

Walker, C. (2005), Postmodernism and nursing science, *The Journal of Theory Construction and Testing*, 9 (1), 5.

Wallace, J., Hunt, J. and Richards, C. (1999), The relationship between organisational culture, organisational climate and managerial values, *The International Journal of Public Sector Management*, 12 (7), 548–64.

Wallis, M. and Tyson, S. (2003), Improving the nursing management of patients in a Hematology/Oncology day unit: an action research project, *Cancer Nursing*, 26 (1), 75–83.

Walshe, K. (2003), Foundation hospitals: a new direction for NHS reform? *Journal of the Royal Society of Medicine*, 96, 106–10.

Walshe, K. and Rundall, T. (2001), Evidence-based management: from theory to practice in health care, *The Milbank Quarterley*, 79 (3), 429–57.

Wanless, D. (2002), *Securing our Future Health; Taking a Long Term View: Final Report*. London: HM Treasury.

Wanless, D. (2004), *Securing Good Health for the Whole Population*. London: HM Treasury/The Stationery Office.

Waring, J. (2004), A qualitative study of the intra-hospital variations in incident reporting, *International Journal for Health Care*, 16 (5), 347–52.

Waterson, J. (2000), Balancing research and action; reflections on an action research project in a social services department, *Social Policy and Administration*, 34 (4), 494–508.

Weber, M. (1968), *Economy and Society*. New Jersey: Bedminster Press.

Webster, C. (1994), The NHS – a kaleidoscope of care – conflicts of service and business values, *British Medical Journal*, 308 (6937), 1172.

Weick, K. and Quinn, R. (1999), Organizational change and development, *Annual Reviews of Psychology*, 50, 361–86.

Westley, F. and Mintzberg, H. (1989), Visionary leadership and strategic management, *Strategic Management Journal*, 10, 17–32.

Wheeler, N. and Grice, D. (2000), *Management in Health Care*. Cheltenham: Stanley Thornes.

Whitehead, D. (2005), Project management and action research: two sides of the same coin? *Journal of Health Organization and Management*, 19 (6), 519–31.

Whyte, W. (1991), *Participatory Action Research*. Newbury Park, CA: Sage Publications.

Wigens, L. (1997), The conflict between 'new nursing' and 'scientific management' as perceived by surgical nurses, *Journal of Advanced Nursing*, 25, 1116–22.

Williamson, G.R. and Prosser, S. (2002a), Illustrating the ethical dimensions of action research, *Nurse Researcher*, 10 (2), 38–49.

Williamson, G.R. and Prosser, S. (2002b), Action research: politics, ethics and participation, *Journal of Advanced Nursing*, 40 (5), 587–93.

Williamson, T. (2005), Work-based learning: a leadership development example from an action research study of shared governance implementation, *Journal of Nursing Management*, 13, 490–9.

Winterton, R. (2004), House of Commons, NHS recruitment and retention debate, 22 June, *Hansard*, column 1307.

Winyard, G. (2003), Doctors, managers and politicians, *Clinical Medicine*, 3 (5), 465–9.

Womack, J., Jones, D. and Roos, D. (1990), *The Machine that Changed the World*. New York: Rawson Associates.

Worthington, F. (2004), Management, change and culture in the NHS: rhetoric and reality, *Clinician in Management*, 12, 55–67.

Wren, D., Bedeian, A. and Breeze, J. (2002), The foundations of Henri Fayol's administrative theory, *Management Decision*, 40 (9), 906–18.

Yeo, R. (2006), Implementing organizational learning initiatives: integrating three levels of learning, *Development and Learning in Organizations*, 20 (3), 10–12.

Young, S. (2002), Evidence-based management: a literature review, *Journal of Nursing Management*, 10, 145–51.

Yukl, G. (2006), *Leadership in Organizations*, 6th edn. New Jersey: Prentice Hall.

Zaner, T. (1968), Action research in management development, *Training and Development Journal*, 22 (6), 28–33.

Zartman, I. (1991), Conflict and resolution: contest, cost and change, *The Annals of the American Academy*, 518, 11–22.

Zuber-Skerritt, O. (2002), A model for designing action learning and action research programs, *The Learning Organization*, 9 (4), 143–9.

Index

Index